GREEN RUBBER BOOTS
A joyful journey to wellness

To Joyce

Bless you!

love

Kathleen Witmer
May 2003

GREEN RUBBER BOOTS
A joyful journey to wellness

Written and illustrated by
KATHLEEN WHITMER

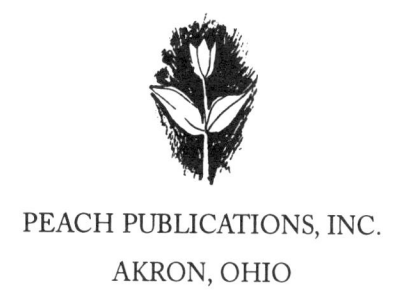

PEACH PUBLICATIONS, INC.
AKRON, OHIO

GREEN RUBBER BOOTS: *A Joyful Journey to Wellness*
Copyright ©1997 by Kathleen Whitmer. All rights reserved. Printed in the United States of America. While the stories are about real people, their names have been changed. No part of this book may be used or reproduced in any manner whatsoever without written permission except in the case of brief quotations embodied in critical articles and reviews. For information address Peach Publications, Inc., 444 Burning Tree Drive, Akron, Ohio 44303.

SECOND PRINTING

ISBN 0–9661079–1–8
ISBN 0–9661079–2–6 (pbk)

Library of Congress Cataloging-in-Production Data:
Whitmer, Kathleen.
Green rubber boots: a joyful journey to wellness/
Kathleen Whitmer. — 1st ed.
p. Cm.

1. Cancer. 2. The National Institutes of Health.
3. Spiritual biography. 4. Whitmer, Kathleen.
5. Self-actualization. 6. Wellness.

97–94485

COVER PHOTOGRAPH
Tulips and Daffodils by the Potomac
oil on canvas
36" x 36"
by Kathleen Whitmer

The original painting is owned by Akron General Medical Center and hangs in The Cancer Center of the Medical Center in Akron, Ohio.

"Happiness is a result of circumstances, but joy endures in spite of circumstances."

Author Unknown

CONTENTS

Preface	i
The Escalator	1
Day of Discovery	5
The Word Cancer	8
The Honors English Teacher	10
The Baby Crib	14
One-Way Ticket	17
The Packed Suitcase	21
Polished Nails	23
The Lobby	26
Man in the Elevator	29
The First Treatment	35
The Parachute	39
The Tulip Dress	42
The Face on the Clock	45
Cemetery Day	49
The Night the Hair Fell Out	53
Funeral Parlor Lady	57
The Neiman-Marcus Lady	62
When It Rains It Pours	65
First Day in My Prosthesis	70
Wine Story	72
Green Rubber Boots	74

Anniversary Dinner 77
The Cigarette Story. 80
The Art Exhibit 83
The Perfect Mouse 87
The Ice Cream Parlor 89
Coon Dog Man 91
Budweiser Man. 95
Not the Measles or the Mumps 97
The Hotel Is Full 102
Taxi Cab Ride. 104
The First Mrs. Whitmer 109
Cancer Lady. 114
Lots of Lasts. 117
The Doctors after Cancer. 122
Retirement 128
Nothing Has to Go Right 130
Amazing Grace. 136
Conclusions 143

With love I wish to dedicate this book to

JERRY, *who never lost faith in me*

and

MARY ANN, ALBERTA, MICHELLE, JEAN

and

EUGENE LINGHAN, S.J.

and

STEVEN ROSENBERG, M.D.

and

WILLIAM LOUGHRY, M.D.

and

CLAUDIA SEIPP, R.N.

and

RACHAEL BROWN, R.N.

and finally

THE PEOPLE OF THE UNITED STATES OF AMERICA

who fund the National Institutes of Health.

PREFACE

After 42 healthy years of what consisted of a normal childhood, success in school, a happy marriage and a rewarding teaching career, I began to notice that the aspirin bottle was always empty and an early flu-like feeling persisted.

Finally, after months of seeing doctors, having tests, and learning more about CAT scans, nuclear medicine and barium than I ever wanted to know, surgery was scheduled.

A grapefruit-sized sarcoma tumor was removed from my vena cava. Sarcoma cancer is cancer of muscle tissue and makes up less than three percent of all cancers. The vena cava is the trunk-like vein that carries blood back to the heart from the lower part of the body. My tumor rested on my liver and pancreas.

For the first time in my adult life I was at home all day, recovering from my surgery. It was the winter of 1979. I had left friends at Kent State University where I taught in the School of Art. I wandered around, I listened, I looked, I pondered, I read, I thought. My dog and my cat listened patiently. The windows of our home were covered with frost.

My surgeon had done his homework. I needed more care if I was to have a chance at living. The National Cancer Institute, one of the fourteen institutes of the National Institutes of Health, was researching sarcoma tumors. Would I lend them my sick body as a clinical study? Would I become a guinea pig?

And so, in April of 1979, a second surgery in Bethesda, Maryland, at the National Institutes of Health, removed a new cancer growth from my vena cava. The Chief of Surgery at NCI removed two pea-sized growths and closed the vein as one might improperly darn a hole in a sock...stitching around the hole and drawing it closed.

I then volunteered for eight weeks of linear radiation and ten months of experimental chemotherapy, which were then administered simultaneously.

The FDA insists on double blind studies. The animals that preceded us in these studies lived across the hall. We could see them in their cages. Their side effects would be our side effects. We saw them come and go. We watched as they were closely monitored.

We were 200 patients, strangers with one thing in common. We all had cancer. Bald... anxious... fearful... happy, we were new friends, we had new surroundings and we were alone but together. The statistics weren't good and the literature didn't lie.

We were all very sick, but we were alive! We laughed, we walked, we joked, we toured museums, we ate ice cream, we discussed illness, wellness, and death. I was the first in our small group to lose my hair. After some coaxing, I showed my bald head. My friend and fellow patient Lucy laughed so hard she fell off her chair onto the old shag-carpeted floor of the government-supported motel where we lived when we weren't in the hospital. Several days later I was able to join in the laughter as Lucy's hair was soon to follow mine!

Today, I enjoy public speaking and the most frequently asked question by myself and others is, Why am I alive?

I don't know for sure. I'd like you to help me decide. Keep in mind I had had two surgeries, chemotherapy, radiation, good care, lots of love and prayers, and I —

- learned to handle stress
- learned to say no and not feel guilty
- learned to behave confidently
- stopped smoking
- learned to avoid uncomfortable situations
- learned to differentiate real fears from irrational fears
- became very verbal with doctors and loved ones, even at the risk of rejection
- learned that I had choices in my life
- learned to put the word "death" in my vocabulary
- learned to eat properly
- learned the connection between good physical health and good mental health, and I
- took complete charge of my life.

I followed and have continued to follow the advice of my doctors... eat lean, eat light, eat clean, and eat fresh.

Today I know that we have far more knowledge than our behavior shows. I work with cancer patients helping to give them the hope that I treasured during my years as a cancer patient. I read, I rest, I laugh, and I think positively.

There are volumes of history within each of these stories, these paragraphs, these sentences. These are stories about the people with whom I lived, the families they left behind in their search for wellness, about their need to help a whole generation of people yet to come, for they knew that their work at the National Institutes of Health was perhaps not going to make them well, but would make their children, or their children's children well.

The stories that evolved from these people as we lived together were stories of life; the realization that death isn't always bad, but life is what happens while you are living. We learned that life and illness are bonding. We learned that good things and bad things are never evenly distributed. You can be at the right place at the right time or you can be at the wrong place at the wrong time. We learned that everyone is a little lonely. We learned that we all cry to be understood. We learned that each of us remains part stranger even to those we love. We learned that the illness of cancer is in a way a terrible illness that isn't necessarily bad. We learned to love one another. To love those around us and the days of being well would be wonderful days, more wonderful than any of the days that preceded our illness.

I could fill books with the cards and letters I received while I was recovering from cancer. Some people gave detailed advice. Others told me of diets that were sure to eradicate cancer cells. Meditation techniques were explained step by step. I even received a prayer cloth with an imprint of a hand that I was to touch. The hand print was the print of a famous contemporary minister. He would heal me if I held my hand on his and asked him to heal me. Most letters, however, expressed anger and shock.

Over and over they asked me, "Why you?"

"Why not me?" I would silently ask myself.

I had had 42 wonderful years. During my stay at the National Institutes of Health, I saw hundreds of children. Their parents wheeled their IV poles beside their strollers.

"Why them?" I would ask. "I have had my chance at life. Their lives have hardly begun."

Is anyone safe? How can we be safe in a universe that is hardly a safe place? Life is unpredictable and sometimes unjust. It seems that some people live long, happy, healthy lives even though society thinks they deserve to suffer, while some people endure one loss after another, though we think they deserve to be blessed. Just like winning and losing the lottery, there is no rhyme or reason to the sadness of some and the happiness of others.

As you read ahead, it is my hope that I will be able to show you that, without the experience of tragedy, we would never know the true gift of life. I thought the world in which I lived before cancer was perfect. Today I realize it was boring. The perfection made me shallow. The days flew by without a hitch. They also flew by without much real gratitude.

Cancer gave me life! The story I want so much to tell after all these years is a story of joy. I do not need to tell you of the horrors of being very sick. I want to share real life experiences, things that actually happened that opened my eyes and the eyes of my cancer mates as we walked together on our path. Through these stories, which are not necessarily in complete chronological order, I want you to walk with us. We dreamed of good health and we learned much during our days the world called "tragic."

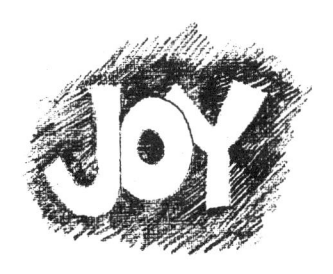

THE ESCALATOR

During the summer of 1978, I felt as though the escalator on which I was riding was changing speeds. One day it would move along as it always had. Then, the next day it would be jerky and unpredictable. My body had always been there and I operated it from within so that I was always outside it. I taught. I painted. I organized my life. I bought groceries, kept a neat, orderly house. That summer felt different. I felt inside myself. When I stepped from the bathtub one evening, I clearly remember having a weird sensation come over me as I dried my body. It felt as though part of me wasn't me.

The area under my right rib cage seemed heavy and bulky.

One warm day as I prepared to attend a wedding shower of a friend, I felt as though the escalator came to stop for just one moment. That little voice inside seemed to whisper to me. I knew that day I had something happening to me that was different from anything I had ever felt before. It was almost as though on that day I stepped completely off the escalator. Everyone else kept moving. Haltingly, I called my doctor. He was a wonderful gentleman. He saw me immediately. But all I could tell him was that I felt funny.

After a series of tests run as an outpatient, I was admitted to the hospital. It was reassuring. He believed me. I had never before been in a hospital. From my window I could see people hurrying in and out the front entrance. They were on that escalator. I was watching it go by. It was a strange new view of life.

The heavy, funny feeling persisted. A group of doctors appeared one morning. A surgeon was in the group. I liked him immediately. We knew and admired some of the same people. The test results showed nothing. They were stumped.

The funny feeling changed into gnawing waves of discomfort that lasted short periods of time. Gradually, the waves became more frequent and lasted longer. One night about 2:00 a.m. I couldn't stand the discomfort. I used my bedside light to beckon a nurse. Each time one came into my room, I really didn't have a specific thing to tell her. I was just in terrible need of someone for something. I was unable to tell them what I really needed.

After three or four times of putting on my light, I heard the heavy heels of sensible work shoes nearing my room. I could hear the sound of nylon stockings rubbing together. It was a sound similar to the sound that kids who wear corduroy pants make. Swish, swish, swish, into my room it came. A sturdy truck-like person stood beside my bed silhouetted against the light of the hall. It felt good having her big body in the room. Maybe she would make the pain go away.

She leaned close to my ear and spoke with her teeth together. "Now, I know women like you. You're enjoying all the attention you are getting from all these men. Now you are not to turn on that light again. We have reports to complete for the morning shift. Do you understand?"

Yes, I understood. There really wasn't anything wrong with me. This professional all dressed in white wearing sensible shoes had said it. Was this feeling I had in my head? Had I made it up? Had I gotten bored and decided to step off the escalator in order to get attention? My life seemed to be on hold. Whatever had I done?

The night was long. I never again put on the light. The next tongue lashing might be worse than the first. I could take no more.

Morning came as it always does. The group of "attention givers" gathered around my bed. They were still mystified. I wondered if they believed me. Maybe they were thinking the same thing the nurse had said in the middle of the night. I found myself hoping they would find something wrong. Better that than having a crazy, imaginative, overactive mind. The surgeon spoke first. He sat on the edge of my bed. He explained that while they all believed I knew my body and that there probably was something going on, they just didn't know what. And so, I was to go home.

Then, just as the rest of the group left the room, he paused and said, "I want you to call me whenever you get one of those waves of discomfort. I don't care when you call. It can be in the morning, at noon, or in the evening."

He will never know what those few words meant to me. I was going home. I was to step back on that jerky escalator but I wasn't going to be alone. I had someone who believed. I had someone to call. I had someone who was going to help me. I wasn't just "one of those women who like all the attention they got from men!"

DAY OF DISCOVERY

Fall quarter 1978 began. The hilly campus was aglow with color. Students were excited about being back on campus. I had three delightful classes. I looked forward to each day. Being with bright, young people is energizing. I tried to feel good. It was work.

Four weeks into the quarter I could no longer stand myself. I could not fight, ignore or deny what was going on inside me. During my morning class break, I called the nice surgeon who had given me permission to call him anytime. He came to the telephone.

At the sound of my voice, he gruffly said, "I want you in my office in thirty minutes."

"Oh, I can't do that. I'm in the middle of teaching a class," I responded.

With that he yelled, "Well, is that damn class more important than your health? Be here in thirty minutes."

He hung up. I swallowed. It was done.

After dismissing my class, I drove to his office. That busy man, the head of the Surgery Department, was waiting for me. It was just like the saying, "If you want something done, give it to a busy person to do." I had struck gold. In the examining room, with all my clothes on, I lay back on the table. His strong knowing hands reached where I pointed.

As his fingers moved under my rib cage he shouted, "Well, Hell, yes, you feel funny. With this big thing pushing on everything, of course, you'd feel funny."

What thing was he referring to? I asked if I could feel it.

He snapped back, "I don't know if you want to."

I assured him that I did. And so that morning I felt for the first time that thing that had been causing me to "feel funny", that thing that had caused those gnawing waves of discomfort. With both hands I reached under my right rib cage and just like a grapefruit, it fell onto the tips of my fingers. I quickly pulled away. The foreign object scared me.

"What is that?" I asked.

"Whatever it is, it's not supposed to be there," he answered.

It was that day, that moment my life changed. I really didn't know then the extent of that change. I just knew things were going to be very different. I drove home with a feeling of relief. Finally, there was something concrete with which to deal. We could now move forward.

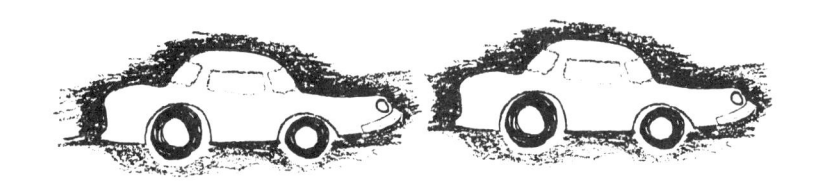

THE WORD CANCER

Once it was determined that a tumor was nestled in the muscle tissue surrounding my pancreas and liver, things moved quickly. The surgery preparation began. I was again admitted to the hospital. Trays holding clear bullion, tea and Jell-o arrived for every meal.

The night before surgery my nurse announced, "We're going to have six enemas."

I asked if we were each going to have three or was she to have five and me one. She was one of those "We" people. I felt as though I were in kindergarten.

"We're going to scrub that colon clean as snow. You never know what they might have to do in there tomorrow."

And so, six enemas later, the soapy water was crystal clear. What an experience "we" went through.

I was wheeled away early the next morning. Several days later, my surgeon, who by now was my hero, came into my room. He usually had five or six young people following close behind. This day there was just one. As he sat on my bed, he placed one big loving hand on my left side. There was a heavy gloom in the air. He really didn't need to say anything. I knew from his face, from his mannerism, from the stillness of his young colleague who stood rigidly on the left side on my bed what he was about to tell me.

After that moment of non-verbal exchange, he quietly and unemotionally stated, "The tumor we removed was malignant. You have cancer."

He patted my hip and told me not to worry. He'd see that I got good care. And so it was over. The words were spoken. The truth was out.

When my husband entered the room minutes after the doctor left, we could only look at one another. There was work to be done. There were plans to be made. The word was out. I had cancer.

THE HONORS ENGLISH TEACHER

Once my first surgery was over and the incision was partially healed, my doctor suggested that I go someplace warm to recover. It was the middle of a freezing cold northeastern winter. Frost and ice covered everything. My husband found a tiny place in Naples, Florida, that we could afford. Once packed, complete with dog and cat, we drove the long drive to the Sunshine State.

The plan was that I would stay for a while to rest and relax and my husband would fly down to see us every other weekend. It seemed like a lovely plan to me. I never had had this kind of freedom.

Gradually my life fell into a nice little routine. Our Irish setter, Kelly, loved her new home and everyone in the neighborhood grew to love her. I was described as "the lady with the pretty red dog".

As I got stronger and stronger, I got braver and braver. Street by street the little cozy town of Naples became my new home. I found bookstores that took old books in return for new ones. Shops were staffed with Northerners who had gotten smart. They each had a snow storm story to tell that had forced them to pack it all up and move to a better life. I have always admired people who are brave enough to take on the risk of their convictions. They knew there had to be some place where they would be happier. They had set out to find it.

My time in Naples was good. I felt strong. My daily visits to the beach, where I sat in a little orange chair at the water's edge, toasted me the color of honey. I wrote letters by the dozens to my friends and my Kent State University colleagues. I was the picture of good health and I had never felt better. Little did I know what was ahead of me. Sometimes it's better not to know.

One beauty of a day, after some time at the beach, I went home happy. I took the dog for her daily walk, poured myself a cool glass of wine and sat down to read my mail. There was a letter from a friend from home, a graduate of a fine Eastern School, and an Honors English teacher. Sally was bright and well-traveled. I was curious to read what was going on at home. I did miss my friends and the familiar surroundings I had grown to love in the 17 years we lived in Akron.

I had never received a letter from Sally. Usually our conversations had been either in person or over the telephone. It would be fun to read her letter.

It began, "All of Akron is talking about your dying".

I read it several times. All of Akron? Talking about my dying? It was a strange vision. Akron is a city of 275,000 people. 275,000 people were talking about me. They were talking about my death.

My immediate reaction was to sit down and write back to her.

My letter began, "I am not dying".

When I looked at that sentence, I realized the silliness of it. Of course I was dying. I had been dying from the day I was born! So was she! The only sad fact is that the bright Honors English teacher from a fancy school in the

East hadn't yet realized her fate and I did. What a wonderful feeling! And, just as I had been dying in wellness, I was dying in illness. It really makes no difference.

If all those 275,000 people had nothing more about which to talk, I was glad I had given them a topic. Maybe it would change their dreams of immortality. The newly-started letter to Sally ended up in the wastebasket and I took Kelly, my red dog, out to cheer up the world.

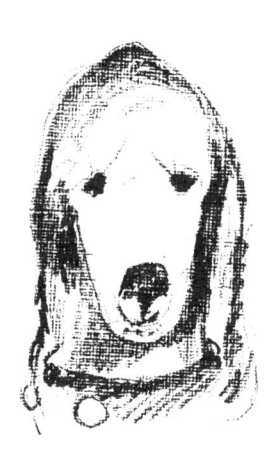

THE BABY CRIB

Upon arrival at the National Institutes of Health, we were taken through a series of tests. Once it was determined that we suited the research study, the expected protocol, or plan, was explained to us in great detail. We were carefully walked through each step. We were taken to the operating room the day before surgery so that the next morning we would be familiar with its color and size. It lessened our anxiety to know what lay ahead.

Irene was to be my nurse after surgery. She showed me where my bed would be in the ICU when I awoke from the anesthetic.

Irene told me her voice would be the first I would hear upon awaking. And, she added that I probably would be annoyed because she would keep talking to get me awake. She assured me that I would be sitting on the edge of my bed by afternoon. Whatever she said was okay with me. I knew I was in good hands.

She carefully pointed out that just across the room, a little to my left, I would see a baby crib. She thought I might be confused by its shape. A three year old child was in that crib. His surgery had been completed the night before. He and his mother were from Florida. She had discovered a lump in his abdomen and had rushed him to the doctor. Upon examining him, the knowledgeable, well-prepared doctor knew the child had a tumor and that it had grown very large and was doubling in size every 24 hours. He knew of the sarcoma study at the National Institute of Health. He called, made all the arrangements, and mother and son were on their way. They never went home to pack or change clothes. The mother sat in the waiting room in her "Florida" bright, light clothing with sandals on her feet. Irene shared with us that when they arrived in Bethesda from Florida in the middle of the night, a crew of doctors and operating room specialists were waiting. In the wee hours of the morning those skilled, heroic people successfully removed a huge tumor from that small child's abdomen. He would not have lived without their dedicated urgency.

When I awoke from my surgery, it gave me great comfort to have that tiny child across from me. Later he was taken from intensive care with a smile on his face into the awaiting arms of his mom who, still in her Florida clothing and sandals, beamed with joy. Her perceptive behavior and good sense and her ability to make quick decisions had saved her child's life!

That child was three. I was 42. That child had lived but three short years.

Seeing all this made me never ask, "Why me?" It made me ask, "Why not me?"

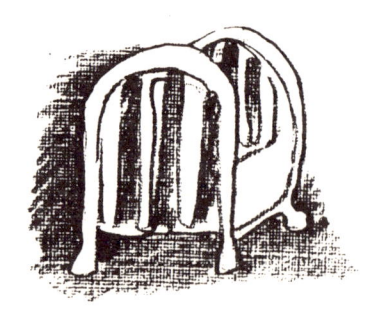

ONE-WAY TICKET

As National Institutes of Health research patients, we were considered government employees. We flew to and from the clinical center in Bethesda, Maryland, on airline government rates. People often ask me about the comings and goings of the process. I sense that most people think that it would be confusing and complicated. They act as though they could never learn the process. It really is quite simple. Let me tell you about it.

Preparing for my trip to the National Institutes of Health, I pictured myself in a camouflage nightgown with a large line of numbers stamped across my chest. I envisioned sleeping on a cot with a scratchy, brindle-colored blanket over me. I was sure they would call me by number. Isn't it strange that we sometimes have a negative image of government institutions? Today I am ashamed of my mistrust of the place that was to save my life.

The first arrangements were made by my doctor. The National Institutes of Health personnel then contacted me. A plane ticket arrived in the mail. A shuttle awaited my arrival at Washington National Airport. A kind gentleman took care of my suitcase. The 45 minute trip through Georgetown and on the beltway that skirts our capital is picturesque and exciting. The van is usually filled with patients traveling to one of the 14 institutes.

Information, laughter and helpful hints were shared during the journey. Upon arrival, we were greeted by Mr. Wing who welcomed us with a big smile. Hundreds of people come and go each year from all over the world, yet he always remembered each of us by name. He has that rare ability of making people feel they are unique, always remembering things from earlier visits. He made sure we got to and from where we needed or wanted to go.

From the beginning, things fell naturally into order. Always called by our first names, the staff, nurses, clinicians and technicians seemed genuinely glad to see us. For me, it has always been like going home. Dedicated people were around every corner concerned about our happiness. It was a place that quite simply practiced the old-fashioned golden rule. They treated us the way they would like to be treated.

Still, that plane ticket which had arrived in the mail a week before the scheduled time of my visit was a one-way ticket. It shocked and scared me.

Questions flashed through my head. Was I ever to return? How long would I be there? Why didn't they know how long I'd be there? Would I ever see home again? Was I going to die in D.C.?

It didn't take long, though, to take comfort in the process, and, once in the main stream of getting well, it all made sense. Of course our return tickets were secured at an in-house travel agency the day before we were released to go home.

Cancer is not a predictable thing. The science of medicine is always changing. Risk-taking can make us anxious. It is, however, one of the essential ingredients of happiness. Reaching into the unknown forces us to leave those old acts of everyday life. As each day goes by, new procedures are discovered, new drugs are produced, and new hope rests in the laboratories that line the National Institutes of Health corridors.

Quite simply, we went home when it was time to go home. We went home in good spirits, with a renewed sense of hope. We went home knowing we were loved.

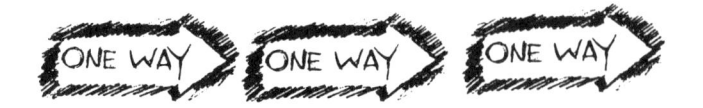

THE PACKED SUITCASE

The night before surgery we were asked to pack our things. The next day our home was to be the operating room. From there, each day was unknown. Government money cannot be spent on empty rooms waiting for patients to return to them. It was an eerie feeling to pack my few personal possessions. Was I ever to see them again? The only thing I was to leave at the end of my bed was a plastic bag holding my toothbrush and some special soap I liked to use on my face. In the quiet of the room, as I lay in bed that suspenseful night, I was filled with the wonder of just how unimportant our things are to us when it really comes down to survival. Stripped of everything, no jewelry, no clothing, no books, no comb or brush, no underwear or pantyhose, we were like newborn babies. We were completely free of the things of the world. It was an uplifting relief! My worries were few. My life was now in the hands of my caregivers and my God. It was a good feeling.

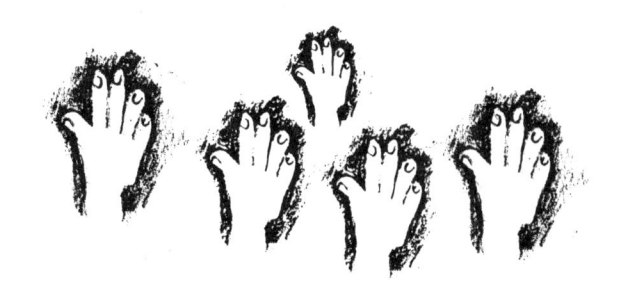

POLISHED NAILS

After surgery and a week in intensive care, I was moved to a "holding tank", a room with four beds directly across from the nurses' station. Later I was moved to a regular hospital room designed to hold two patients. I found that my possessions had been unpacked for me. I hung my legs over the side of the bed. I was unplugged from all the tubes and machines. I felt free and wonderfully new. I opened the top drawer of the small dresser beside my bed. Carefully placed within were the few things I had brought.

"Oh, look," I said to myself, "nail polish."

I had forgotten that I had brought it. Why had I brought it? I seldom had ever had polished nails. Having been an art teacher all my life, my hands always looked terrible. Days in clay, paint, plaster and the materials of an art room had taken their toll. When I looked into my lap, it was fun to see for the first time rested hands with clean fingernails and a little length.

I reached for the forgotten polish and ever so carefully, I painted each nail. That was my first big task since my surgery. Exhausted, I lay back on the clean, crisp, white pillow pleased with my accomplishment.

I placed my hands carefully on top of the blanket and sheet. Wet finger nails, if left to dry under the blanket resembled little waffles. The weave of the blanket pressed into the wet enamel makes a lovely texture, but not a texture complimentary to the finger nail.

With my nails carefully drying and my eyes closed, resting from my work of the day, I heard the voices of my doctor and his team of doctors, interns, research nurses and social workers. I could feel them assembled around my bed.

I was about to open my eyes when, Gretchen, my social worker, announced, "Oh, look, her nails are polished!"

My eyes popped open. I was delighted that she had noticed. I smiled.

Gretchen then inquired, "Who painted them?"

I proudly replied, "I did."

"Why?" she asked.

Why had I painted my nails? Was it because the polish was there or because I needed red nails or because it just seemed the thing to do. I wasn't sure. I was alive. It felt good to do things again.

In her report, years later I discovered what she had written concerning my behavior… "Kathleen polished her nails today. She is still in denial concerning her illness."

Be careful when you polish your nails, for around some corner there might be someone critically judging the why's of such simple behavior.

What seems natural to someone getting well can easily be misunderstood by people who have been blessed with good health.

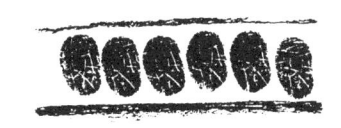

THE LOBBY

During the times we did not have to be hospitalized, we spent our National Institutes of Health days living in a little motel chosen by the government. It was one of those places you see as you drive down the main street in any city. You probably have asked yourself, "Who stays in a place like that?"

The lobby had thread-bare carpet, two chairs and two couches. The fabric on the chairs and couches was dark with oil stains from the hands of people who had used them over the years. That furniture made me realize why my mother had used those arm covers on our furniture when I was a child. Cover removal was only for company. Then and only then were the covers tucked under the sofa cushions to be returned the minute company left.

Also, in the entrance of our "home away from home" were several huge plastic plants. Every leaf was covered with an inch of dust. Like children with frosted car windows, we often wrote our initials on the dusty leaves. One day we took delight in scrubbing each leaf with some sudsy water.

Tourists looking for a place to spend the night often stopped. They would walk in the door with big smiles on their faces and then, in spite of the dusty plastic plants, the threadbare carpet and the darkened fabric on the arms of the furniture, they walked over to the desk to check in. Gradually, they would glance at the group of us clustered together sharing how our day had gone, and then their necks would snap back in a double take. One would elbow the other and, predictably, they would tell Judy, the desk clerk, not to bother. The dust, the plastic plants, and the oldness, they were willing to overlook; but, our bald heads, wigs, scarves, caps, pale coloring, my broken leg, others' amputated arms and legs made them run. They didn't want to look at us and they surely didn't want to catch whatever we had! If they had decided to stay, they would have realized more fully the realness of life. It's not easy being sick in a society that worships wellness.

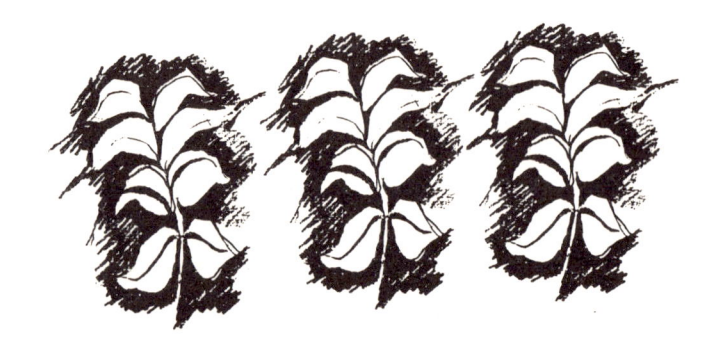

MAN IN THE ELEVATOR

Radiation has a mystery to it. There is nothing, yet there is something. With surgery, I could see the remaining scar; I could understand the process. And, with chemotherapy, I could see the liquid drug travel from the syringe into my vein. I understood its path and its mission.

Radiation was different. It was to start just two weeks after I had been bombarded with surgery and chemotherapy. My tolerance for more abuse was at an all time low. Trying to be a good patient, I reported to an assigned room where a lady drew a "map" on the front right-hand side of my abdomen. I rolled over and she drew a similar "map" on my back directly behind the map on the front of my body. She carefully measured using information from my chart; which she cautiously checked as she worked. She used an indelible blue marking instrument. When I looked in the mirror the first time after the "maps" had been drawn, I saw a rectangular shape both front and back. The corner lines crossed one another. She told me not to use soap on the lines and told me to report back should the lines fade or disappear. I was told to avoid creams and to wear cotton next to my body.

From there, I was told to report to the Radiation Department. The elevator had a B3 button. Radiation was in the basement. It was an area away from everything and everyone. I have often wondered how people work in such an area. The machines obviously had to be buried in the bowels of the building so they would not expose healthy people to the dangers of radiation.

My doctor was a small and obviously brilliant man. Using layman's language, he tried to explain the radiation process to me. I have never really completely understood how it all worked. I was, however, receptive and responsive.

Each morning for eight weeks, I was to report to the radiation area. Twenty to thirty of us sat around the outside walls of the room waiting our turn. The room had a large square table in the center cluttered with magazines. The room was dark, a difficult room in which to read. Of course, there were no windows. The carpet and furniture were dark brown. There were no plants. There was nothing soft.

None of us had a appointment for a specific time. Our radiation therapists called us by the order of the area that needed radiation. Patients receiving radiation to their heads usually went first. Then they moved the setting of the machine down. And so, we were called in order of the position of the area on our bodies that needed radiation. This process helped them work more efficiently; they didn't have to move the machine from top to bottom and back again.

The room with the magical machine was large and cold. A long metal examining-like table was in the center. The heavy, bulky and complicated machine hovered over the table. There were spaces in the table that could be removed so that the beams of linear radiation could hit the exact rectangular "maps" that were drawn on my body. Once I was in exactly the right spot lying with the area to be radiated over the grid-like tennis racquet area of the table, the eye of the linear accelerator was pulled down about a foot from my body. Then, the therapist left the room. Behind her she slammed a huge metal gate-like door that bolted from the outside.

I lay very still in the dark cold room on the metal table with the hole in it.

Then the voice of the therapist came through a speaker someplace in the room, "Radiation will begin. Lie very still. Do not move. Hold your breath."

The machine hummed a flat even sound. The head of the machine then rolled over and around the table so that it was positioned under the table aiming its beam exactly where the map was drawn on my back. The invisible mystery went through my body from front to back and then from back to front. Cancer cells in its path were destroyed along with some healthy cells. And, a year after the procedure, my right kidney no longer appeared on any test. It also had been zapped.

It was all a weird and puzzling process. So, while chemotherapy was eating up bad cells along with good ones, so was the radiation. Neither could tell the difference. It was an exhausting way to begin each day. To this day, I'm not sure if the exhaustion came from the trauma of the paralyzing process or the actual radiation. The waiting sometimes seemed endless; the third floor basement was lonely and segregated. The sadness of the time, along with the humming machine, was unnerving. Our caregivers who wore heavy quilted metal shields to protect themselves from the radiation worked methodically.

My first day riding down the three floors on the elevator was scary. The unknown awaited me. There was a tall, thin man in the elevator with me. He must have sensed my apprehension. He asked if it was my "first time". His voice was barely audible. He saw my fear. When I replied that yes, it was an all-new experience for me, he proceeded to warn me not to let them burn me up the way they had him. With that, he held back his shirt collar and exposed a bright red, heavily scarred neck. His speech had obviously been involved in the mutilation. My fear now turned to horror.

The nice technician noticed my obvious, fearful behavior. On the verge of tears, I told her about my conversation with the gentleman in the elevator. Her eyes widened and then she put her arm around me. It felt reassuring. She knew the man of whom I spoke.

She told me his story. He had had cancer twenty years before. He had been treated at another hospital with a radiation machine that had been obsolete years ago. He represented the results from an earlier era in cancer treatment.

I learned a real lesson that first day of radiation and have continued to remind myself and others that we must be careful to whom we listen during such a fragile time in our lives. I have found that everyone has a cancer story. They have an aunt, an uncle, a friend or a neighbor who has had cancer. Then they start through the grueling details. Someplace along the way, I realized that the words of these well-meaning people simply had to go in one ear and out the other.

We are as different in illness as we are in wellness. Just as there are no two fingerprints that are the same, there are no two cancers exactly the same; nor are there reactions to or from any of the procedures going to be the same. The man in the elevator scared me to death; but, at the same time, he taught me an invaluable lesson. For, I learned that, "fear makes the wolf bigger than he is." (author unknown). I'm glad it happened early into my treatment. It was a good experience. From that day on, I became a patient and compassionate listener but I never internalized others' illnesses. Mine was my very own. I also re-learned what my Irish mother had taught us as children that "if you can't say something good or something positive, it's better not to say anything at all".

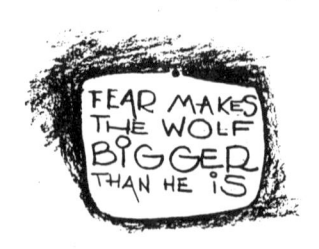

THE FIRST TREATMENT

The unknown can cause us great anxiety. The morning I was to have my first chemotherapy was long and syncopated with sounds and moves done mechanically like a toy soldier wound too tightly.

The room had 12 beds, six along each wall. Mine was beside the window. It was a warm, sunny day and people sat out in the grass eating their lunches. Some ate from brown bags, others from cafeteria trays. The view reminded me of an updated painting by Surat, **Picnic by the Sea.**

Lucy, who was in the bed next to me, was the first to get the experimental drug. I was to be next. My husband, Jerry, sat beside my bed reading. His knuckles were white as he clenched his book.

My doctor and his team of excited interns and fellows came to my left side. "Are you ready?"

"As ready as I'll ever be," I replied.

Each step of the procedure was explained to me detail by detail. Needles flushed, the site prepared, the experimental drug was unwrapped from its' dark, gray cloth covering. The syringe looked like one from a child's toy doctor's bag. It was oversized and filled with what looked like catsup. I watched as the Adriamycin slowly entered my body through the thin needle. It was years before I could look at a bottle of catsup without having my stomach do a flip flop.

I was to tell those monitoring the procedure what I was feeling. The mice that preceded us in the study couldn't talk to them. I felt the catsup-like juice travel into my body. I could feel it as it went down my arm and into my blood stream. As it moistened the tissue of my nose, I felt a stinging feeling, and, as it traveled through my eye area, involuntary tears ran down my cheeks. As it went through my heart, I felt as though a tiny army of men wearing rubber boots were marching in unison.

Midway into my first treatment, a young doctor stood at my bedside listening to my descriptions. Suddenly, I realized I had started my period that morning. Innocently I asked if the chemotherapy would affect my menstrual cycle.

"Oh," he announced joyfully, "that's the last one of those you'll ever have."

Wow! In that list of side effects, had I neglected to read something so important?

"No, it wasn't on the list," I was haphazardly told.

I lay there for a minute thinking of the consequences. I had just gone through menopause! Sadly, I felt a bit of anger.

"Do you suppose if this drug shortened a man's penis by three inches, it would be included in the list of side effects?" I asked.

The young doctor's eyes widened. He was obviously embarrassed.

He left my bedside and I heard him repeat our conversation to my oncologist from whom I heard a hearty laugh.

In no time, he was at my bedside. He was apologetic and in complete agreement.

Several years later, it was rewarding for me to meet a young lady, who, upon reading the updated list of side effects, chose to postpone her chemotherapy. She wanted to see if she could have the child she had always dreamed of having. Ten months after having had a pelvindectomy, she was able to carry and deliver a full term, beautiful baby girl. She was then "ready" for her chemotherapy!

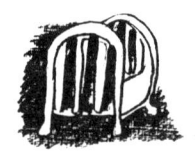

THE PARACHUTE

Once the eight weeks of radiation was completed, I was permitted to return to Akron. With two rounds of chemotherapy, surgery, and radiation behind me, it was good to get home. With seven more treatments of chemotherapy ahead, each spaced 28 days apart, I marked the dates on the calendar. It was frightening to leave the constant, careful monitoring I had grown to appreciate as my life line to living. While going home had, of course, been my goal, it was, at the same time frightening. I was going to be alone; away from my caregivers.

From those monthly visits, I was moved to bi-monthly visits. After that period of time passed, I was gently moved to visits every three months. When I had begun this walk to wellness, I dreamed of the day when I would graduate. Yearly check-ups were my goal. What a celebration it would be! Just think, after what seemed to be hundreds of trips filled with anticipation and anxiety, we would have all those behind us. I was sure that day would be a day of celebration. It would certainly call for something special.

A strange thing started to happen during these back and forth trips. Our trip to the Cleveland airport is a 25 minute drive. In anticipation of what lay ahead, I would get a lump in my stomach, my mouth would become dry, I would hear my heart beating in my ears. That all happened 18 years ago. To this day, a trip to the airport brings back all those same feelings. The impending experience was so intense it left a lasting imprint on my consciousness.

For several years, I returned every six months.

On one of those visits, my doctor announced, "Well, Kathleen, I think you are out of the woods".

Wow, what I had dreamed about was actually happening. It was hard to believe.

He then added, "You need only to return once a year for a follow-up."

Could I be hearing correctly? Had it really happened?

Then instead of the anticipated feeling of joy, I felt this sinking feeling. I was being cut free. I could fly on my own. The cancer was gone. I glanced out the window and felt as though I had been nudged from the airplane without my parachute.

Cancer makes us dependent souls. We work to get from CT scan to CT scan. Not a day passes we don't wonder, "Will today be the day it returns?" Gradually, the feeling subsides. The everyday tasks start to take over and flying is wonderful. Yes, flying alone is more wonderful than it ever was before the disease.

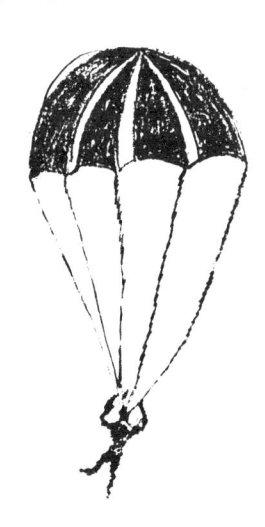

THE TULIP DRESS

Nausea can be debilitating. Is there anything worse? The wondering, the "what if's" and the unknown can cause anxiety. When we finished receiving our chemotherapy, we were sent home with a pile of plastic-lined bags to have just in case we needed them. I was given a drug called Compazine. It was a small, seemingly harmless yellow pill. It was designed to prevent the chemotherapy from causing waves of nausea. I was a novice. I hadn't a clue what was going to happen or how I would react.

The Compazine seemed to work. That evening I was able to accompany my husband to dinner. I nursed a cup of tea. I sat very still. I couldn't look at any of the food in the dining room. The catsup bottle on the next table looked like a big red monster. It was years until I could eat it again. Just the sight of it would trigger a tumble in my stomach.

That evening, with my first chemotherapy under my belt, I fell asleep easily. And then it started. As if I had been given some horrible hallucinating drug, I dreamed bright colorful, out of body dreams that took me to weird places. I zoomed about the room in mid-air. My skin left my body. I stood in a corner of the room opposite our bed watching myself sleep. There I was, watching from afar as I slept peacefully.

I can remember perfectly being completely separated from that person in the bed. We were the same person but there were two of us. And, a little confused by it all, I remember looking down only to see that I was wearing a bright yellow dress. It had two long green-stemmed red tulips appliqued on the front.

It was the dress that Aunt Mame had bought me to wear to school the first day of first grade. How I loved it! It felt good wearing it again.

I awoke the following morning exhausted from the adventures of my dreams. I felt my skin. I checked to see that it was all in place. It was back on my body. My yellow dress with the lovely red tulips was gone, replaced by the soft white cotton nightgown I had worn to bed.

While the Compazine had kept the nausea to a minimum, it also had had serious side effects. When I told the story of the yellow tulip dress to my doctor, he laughed. He was interested in hearing the detailed memory of my "trip".

We both agreed that Compazine was obviously not the drug to use for my nausea. And so, like always, I was listened to and praised for being able to give such detailed feedback. To prevent nausea in the future, I was given a drug called Thorocan. From that time on, I had very little nausea and there was no more wearing the lovely yellow dress with the red tulips. It was packed away forever!

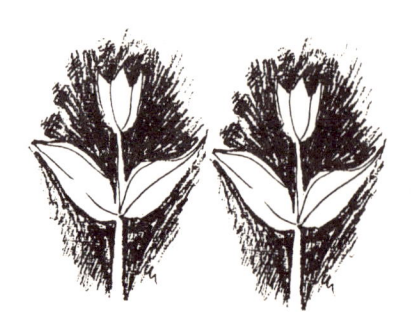

THE FACE ON THE CLOCK

An exciting part of any extended medical problem is the witnessing of the great changes in technology. I laugh as I remember that first barium enema. Today, the test has gone from "intolerable" to "almost okay".

The day before the test unnerved and overwhelmed me. The night before had been horrendous. Various things I drank caused the expected results. The morning of the test was to measure my endurance over the uncomfortable.

At eight a.m. I arrived at the barium enema area for my new experience. I was asked to change to the usual hospital gown that flies open in the back. I sat on a long, cold bench along a corridor wall. Others joined me. Quietly we sat, too anxious to speak to one another. Finally, I was next. I had moved to the head of the line. We were given a milk shake cup filled with a chalk-like drink. After downing one cup, two more followed. I was stuffed to the brim. I then lay on a cold stainless steel table. A plastic bag filled with barium hung on an apparatus beside the table like a heavy bag of liquid white plaster.

All that liquid was to become part of me. My abdomen grew larger and larger as my colon swelled with the white chalk.

Once the bag was emptied, the technician used what resembled a thin wooden board used to remove pizzas from the oven to paddle my stomach pushing the barium into place. The doctor appeared and began his work. I was asked to roll from side to side, and the table flopped up and down, end to end. The doctor delighted in his task.

I heard him say, "Beautiful pictures!"

In agony, I fought the need to expel the barium. I glanced around the room. The brown linoleum rim around the institution floor was spotted with barium. The nurse kept encouraging me.

"You can hold it," she assured me.

When I pointed out the spots of barium around the room, she did admit that some people just couldn't hold it. Would I be one of them?

Finally, the doctor finished. I asked him whatever made him select this speciality. Can you imagine ever falling in love with your "barium enema doctor"?

Now, for the crowning glory of the morning. The technician ordered, "Now just lie there for a few minutes while I go develop your pictures."

There I was alone, filled with barium in that barium-spattered room on that cold table. My body was rigid. The large clock stared at me from overhead. The second hand clicked loudly. Click, click, click.

When would she return? How long was "a few minutes"? Where had she gone to develop the pictures, leaving me ready to explode? Would I add to the spattered walls?

The clock seemed to sneer down at me. How could a few minutes seem so long? The clock became my enemy. It clicked, clicked, clicked ever so smugly.

She returned. The pictures were perfect. I had made it!

Today, the test has changed dramatically. A little barium is inserted along with a little air and an inflated balloon secures the barium. Technology has taken this horrid experience and made it "bariumable".

CEMETERY DAY

During the year of my chemotherapy, I was able to be at home on Mother's Day. It was a beauty of a day. Warm sunshine greeted us. When my husband, Jerry, asked what I'd like to do for the day, I suggested we go visit the grave of his brother who had died the year before.

"You want to visit the cemetery on Mother's Day?" he asked, puzzled.

I think he thought that I was joking.

My mother had died with no plans for the inevitable. On January 2, 1972, we stood up to our knees in snow looking for a place to bury our beloved Lucy Casey. Would the tree overhead really ever have leaves? What did the grass look like? I decided that cold day in 1972 to never let this happen to those I love.

And so, off to the cemetery we went, under the guise of visiting Jerry's brother, Clair. Once there, I suggested that we should see if we could select our own final resting place.

"Buy cemetery lots on Mother's Day? There won't be anyone working today," Jerry exclaimed.

Since it was my idea and he was sure no one would be in the little office building, he jokingly had me run up to the office to see if anyone was working.

I had fallen several months into my chemotherapy treatment and had broken my ankle. That day I had a cast to my knee on my right leg. I hobbled up the few steps, opened the door and was greeted by a huge, heavy-set man surrounded by a desk filled with papers all askew and buried in a cloud of smoke from the cigarettes he was chain smoking. His ashtray ran over with the ugly, smelly remains.

In a hurry to get out of the place, I innocently announced, "My husband wants to buy me a Mother's Day present."

Now you must remember, there I stood bald, with a cast on my leg. The gentlemen looked up and his face quickly told me he thought he should hurry and get his map out of his desk drawer.

I had him mark places in the old section that were under trees. I wanted to know who my neighbors were going to be, and I like shade. He circled some areas in red on the little map he handed me. We drove from one area to the next. We got out of the car at each place and agreed that we didn't like the view. We finally rounded a corner and there it was...a beauty of a piece of land. Nestled under a tree, the space could hold ten people. I have always hated crowds. The view was wonderful. The tree was old and large and it shaded the entire area. What a find!

The following Christmas, Jerry took me to do a little Christmas shopping. As we walked through Saks Fifth Avenue, we ran into two friends from home. Lois and I had been teachers together and we always had much to talk about. Jerry and Oliver had been friends for a long time.

As I listened to Lois, I overheard Jerry saying, "I'm not buying her anything for Christmas; she hasn't used her Mother's Day gift yet!"

That was 17 years ago, and my gift remains unused. There are times I threatened Jerry that he might be the first to use the gift!

Being prepared for even the worst in life isn't a bad idea. It is comforting to know that job is behind us.

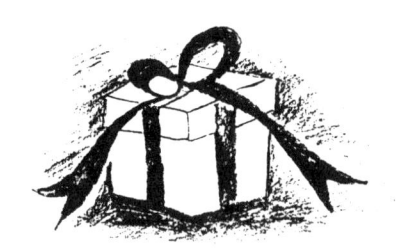

THE NIGHT THE HAIR FELL OUT

In preparing us for what was ahead in our protocol, we were permitted to see some of the mice that preceded us in our research study. All the mice were carefully reproduced at a place not far from the National Institutes of Health. They were delivered in cages and stacked neatly outside the research center. It was an ominous sight. Those perfect little creatures were carefully singled out one to a cage. Each cage was labeled, and each label told the date of birth, weight and size. The labels included who their parents had been. We could walk down the research corridors and see them in their laboratory studies. Their side effects would be our side effects.

Along with the list of information concerning the side effects of this experimental drug we were to receive was, of course, the dreaded fact that we were to lose our hair. Not only were we told we would lose it, but they even told us the exact day it would come out. Ten days after our first treatment "it" would happen. We were told to prepare for it. A prescription was written for our visit to the wig store. We were to get our prosthesis at a nice little wig shop down the beltway not far from Bethesda. A taxi took us to and from the shop.

That day is vivid in my memory. There was this "I'm doing this but I'll probably never need it" attitude about my behavior. The human spirit is a wonderful thing. Sometimes we protect ourselves from what we just aren't ready to accept by telling ourselves, "not me". I was sure that my thick, heavy, salt and pepper hair would never fall out. Heavens, it was far different hair from the hair I had seen on those little mice!

At the wig shop, a nice lady helped me. There was a beautiful red wig on display. Instantly, I reached for it. Oh, I had always wanted to be a redhead. My Grandma Glenny was a redheaded Irish lass straight from County

Clare. Everyone in the shop was excited at what a wonderful redhead I would make.

But, I realized I would eventually go home to a city already abuzz about my illness. I just couldn't imagine giving them more to talk about. I finally purchased the ugliest salt and pepper thing you ever saw. With my own hair under it to hold it in place, it wasn't too bad. I was ready for the big event that was surely never to happen.

As I sat at the little white Formica desk in my small government-provided room one evening, my head started to tingle. It felt just like a scab I once had on my knee as a child just before the scab fell off. As I reached up to scratch that little tingle, my hand filled with hair. The white Formica surface was covered with hair. Panic went through me. My hair was falling out; all of it was falling out. Like removing hat after hat, I took handfuls of hair from my head. I placed it in the cream colored plastic waste basket under the desk. It was filled to the brim when I finished. It was hard to believe that my head had held all that hair!

I paced back and forth, taking in deep breaths of cool air. Now I had to look for the first time at my bald head. Mother had always told me that I was born a beautiful bald baby. How I longed to have her here to tell me the same thing!

And so, like when we watch a scary movie, I put my hands to my face, separated my fingers, and peeked through the little openings. Gradually, I was able to absorb more and more. It was, indeed, gone. Whatever was to come next? Just then the telephone rang. It was my husband, Jerry.

He cheerfully asked, "What's new?"

Yes, we can protect ourselves by denying. But, eventually we must accept the truth. Then, and only then, can we move forward.

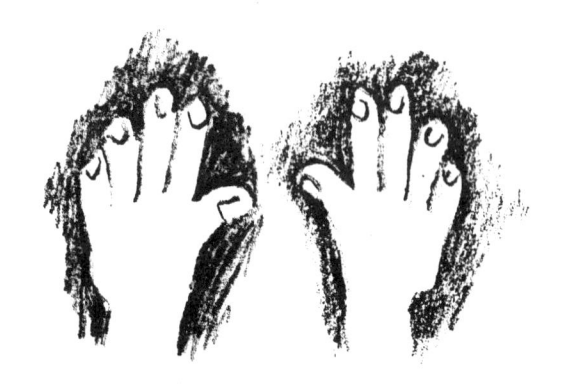

FUNERAL PARLOR LADY

Facing the world the morning after my hair fell out was traumatic. I got up early. I worked hard to make myself as presentable as possible. I selected all my favorite articles of clothing to wear from the few things I had brought from home.

I was a 42 year old woman with a bald head. If I had been a baby or a grown man it would have been acceptable. A bald baby is cute and Yul Brenner probably made a fortune being bald.

I shyly gathered with the other patients in the lobby waiting for the shuttle. It was a pleasant, cool, sunshiny morning. Cheerful words were exchanged. We boarded the bus. I was in the front aisle seat beside a nice lady I had seen a few times but had never spoken with.

I was bursting to tell someone about how my hair had fallen out the night before. I was anxious to tell someone how I took handsful of hair from my head and placed them in the little plastic wastebasket beside the desk where I performed this gruesome task.

And so, I blurted out the honest, horrible truth, "All my hair fell out last night."

There, someone knew! I guess the fact that she had an obvious plastic wig placed crookedly on her shiny head made it easier to tell her. She was a good listener. She showed concern as I described the ordeal. I told her how I had to peek through my fingers to take that first look at my new head. I was like a child at a frightening movie. After years of viewing the expected image, I had to peek, not sure of what I was to see.

Hair by the handsful fell out. Where had all that hair been? When the task was completed, the wastebasket was full. As I told my story, I felt better. Sharing can be a kind of therapy. Her clear brown eyes told me she understood. She was silent.

And, when I was finished telling my story, she asked one simple question. "What did you do with the hair in the wastebasket?"

I looked blankly into her plain face. What had I done with those handsful of dead hair that I had removed like taking many hats off my head? The image of the filled wastebasket flashed into my mind.

"I threw it away", I replied.

"You threw it away?" she responded with alarm. "You threw it away, all of it?"

Thoughts raced through my mind. Had I not listened? What had my caregivers told me to do with it? With my artistic spirit, I have often been told that I don't listen carefully enough. Pictures form quickly as people speak to me. Had I not done the right thing? I searched my brain trying to remember what I had been told to do with the dead hair. Finally, sure that I had made a serious error, I gathered myself up and was about to ask the driver to stop so that I could get off the shuttle to return to my room in order to retrieve the hair from the plastic wastebasket.

As I stood, not looking forward to my walk back to the hotel, I quickly asked my friend, "What did you do with yours?"

She replied, "I put it in a zip-lock bag."

She moved her fingers in such a way as to demonstrate the zipping of the carefully sealed bag just as it is done in the television commercials. I wondered where I was going to get a zip-lock bag. And then, one final question occurred to me.

I asked, "Why?"

And, as she threw back her shoulders proudly and clung to her worn, brown, heavy duty handbag she replied, "To give to my funeral parlor director."

Wow, to give to her funeral parlor director!

I sat back down. There was silence. I was glad it was almost time to get off the shuttle bus. I didn't know what to say. Never in a hundred years had this notion occurred to me. I was a living person in the process of getting well. I was living with cancer. I would have a beautiful new head of hair again soon. This was temporary.

Today as I think about this experience, I wish I had asked just one more question. I have wondered and pondered just how she thought her funeral parlor director was going to get each piece of that dead hair back onto her head. Do you suppose she thought he was going to glue it piece by piece? Would he use Elmer's glue or rubber cement? Or, do you suppose he was going to put glue on her head and dunk it in the hair as we dunk an ice cream cone in chocolate bits? Whatever her answer, I decided that day that I was living with cancer, she was dying with it.

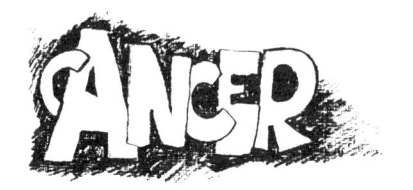

THE NEIMAN MARCUS LADY

Solving "the bald head problem" became a real challenge. I had this terrible need to tell everyone I saw what was about to happen to me. One day I walked to the Neiman Marcus store that was a few blocks down Wisconsin Avenue. I knew there would be people there who might be sympathetic to my plight. The people of Bethesda knew of the research hospital up the street built on 350 acres of land. They were patient listeners. As I admired a purple silk blouse with a high neck, a lovely young woman offered to wait on me. Somehow I thought that if the neck of the blouse was high, it would help to hide my bald head. Now, wasn't that silly?

When I told the saleslady my story, she took charge. She escorted me to a large fitting room and told me she'd be back in a few minutes. As I sat there, I wondered what she might be up to. She returned just as she said she would, loaded with lovely scarves, earrings and a variety of "bald head problem solvers". She was one of those women who could buy everything she wore at the Goodwill and come out looking like a million dollars. She had that skill of combining colors, patterns, and shapes and of knowing how to fold and tie in such a way that things look like they do on movie sets. She wound a beautiful soft paisley scarf around my head, warning me to never use silk because it wouldn't stay put on a bald surface. She tucked rumpled tissue paper under it and tied it behind my right ear. I was transformed! Big earrings filled in the empty spaces. She then took me to the cosmetic counter where she taught me the art of eye makeup. The first time I looked in the mirror it reminded me of the old song "You Gotta Accent the Positive, Eliminate the Negative".

She advised me to go out and catch the TR6 bus, ride it a few blocks and then ride it back to the hotel. I was to watch for the reactions of the people. Wow! Much to my surprise, I discovered that most people were so wrapped up in themselves, where they were going and who they were with, that they really didn't notice how I looked. The people who did notice smiled positively, seeming to think I was smart for having my hair pulled back under a cool scarf on such a sticky, hot D.C. day. Little did they know!

Thank God for the Neiman Marcus lady. She surely helped to solve my "bald head problem" in a creative, refreshing way. A year later, when I finally had a new head of hair ready for the world to see, I sadly tucked all my lovely scarfs away. They had been good friends to me.

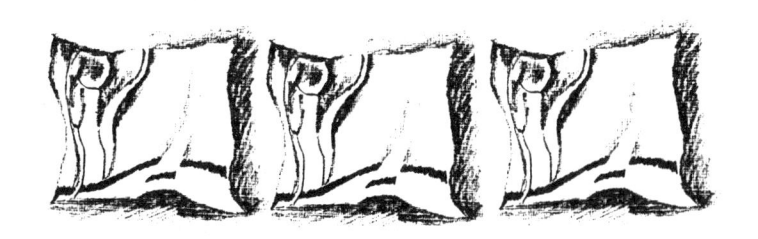

WHEN IT RAINS IT POURS

Our protocol called for us to have chemotherapy every 28 days. The evening prior to my third treatment, I went out to dinner with a lovely lady from San Francisco. She was the wife of a cancer patient who had been admitted to the hospital earlier in the week. He was having serious problems handling some of the chemicals he was taking to quiet his cancer cells.

Louise and I liked one another the moment we met. Around 6:00 p.m. we took a cab three blocks down Wisconsin Avenue to a charming little French restaurant. Because I was to have my third chemotherapy treatment the following day, I had a small green salad. I tried not to concentrate on what the next day had in store. I did, however, know enough to eat a light dinner. It was to be a quiet, peaceful evening. Tomorrow was important.

We left the restaurant after our enjoyable time together and set out to get a cab. I had watched my husband flag a cab many times. It was easy. You simply held up your arm, waved it about and a cab stopped close to the curb. Since I was younger than my new friend, I took it upon myself to flag the taxi. As I raised my arm, I took one big step. I didn't look down. Just as I went into the street, I tumbled over the uneven handicapped curbing. Before I knew what had happened to me, I was on the ground. The tires of the taxi were next to my nose. It was a close one. The driver and my friend showed real concern.

"Are you okay?"

Not wanting to be a problem, I assured them I was fine even though my leg, ankle and foot really did hurt.

Isn't it funny that, when we were children and we fell, we reacted honestly? We cried. We looked to see what hurt and we ran to someone to take our hurt away. We even wanted someone to kiss the bruised area. As adults, we fall but we quickly get up as though nothing happened, feeling awkward and stupid. We deny there could be anything wrong and we dismiss any help from others. I wouldn't even allow myself to look at what was throbbing with pain.

We left the taxi, said our farewells, and went to our rooms. Once in my room I undressed and showered. I still ignored my right leg. The warm water would wash away the pain. I soaped and scrubbed. And then I stepped from the shower and attempted to dry myself. As I moved down my body, I finally had to look at my right ankle and foot. They were twice the size of my left foot and ankle.

"Mercy, what have I done?" I wondered.

How could this happen? I had to be in tip-top shape for tomorrow. What should I do? My mind zoomed from one thing to another. It was eleven o'clock; I was alone. Whom should I call? Isn't it strange how, even though we may never have broken anything, we know immediately when something is really broken?

I stared at the swollen, throbbing foot. I prayed that it would just go away. Wishing would make it happen. I was wrong. I needed more than prayer. I needed help.

Suddenly the face of Miss Black, the head nurse on the surgery floor who had cared for me after my surgery, came to me. I picked up the telephone. She was there. She was concerned.

She told me, "Stay put. Someone will come for you."

I finally accepted the inevitable. I dressed and waited for help to come.

The driver carefully delivered me to the front door of the clinical center where one of the doctors on duty waited with a wheelchair. He took me to a sleepy x-ray area. A yawning technician turned on the lights, cranked up his machine and within minutes I knew for sure that I had a broken foot.

What a mess I was in. No hair. No pajamas. No toothbrush. No nothing.

So, exhausted and exasperated, I was put into a clean, comfortable bed on the surgery floor where I had been cared for just two months before. Comforted with ice on my foot, I was told not to worry. Tomorrow was another day.

First thing the next morning, after more x-rays, a physician from a hospital in Washington, D.C. arrived to set my foot since this kind of treatment is not done at the

National Institutes of Health. He created a plaster cast up to my knee.

That afternoon I was taken in a wheelchair to the chemotherapy room. What a sorry sight I was! That day I had to try to learn to use crutches in between bouts of nausea from the Adriamycin.

When it rains, it does pour, doesn't it? But God seems always to give us a strong umbrella to face the wind and the rain. Hold on tightly and the storm will subside and the sun will come out again.

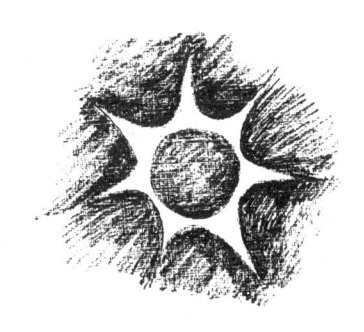

FIRST DAY IN MY PROSTHESIS

Bald heads were never made for wigs. My neck got stiff making sure I didn't make a move that would be too quick for the wig. The plastic was rough on my tender new "out for the first time" head. The humid Washington, D.C. weather made the wig unbearable. My first day in it was like that first day of wearing Kotex and a sanitary belt, only worse. At least the whole world couldn't see that.

After a day of wearing the wig, I returned to my room. My hand shook as I went to unlock my door. That manmade, plastic, pretend thing on my head had tortured me for as long as I could stand it. When I went to take it off, it was just like removing a suction cup from a window. That was to be the last day for that! There had to be a better solution to the problem.

Much later when I returned home, our cat, Sparky, found that wig and was sure it was some terrible animal that had come from somewhere in my suitcase to harm him. He immediately pounced on it and ripped it to pieces. Good Sparky!

The best solution to a problem is not always the first solution.

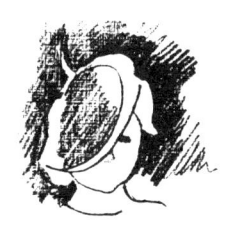

WINE STORY

When all my radiation treatments were completed, I was asked to stop in to see the Director of the Department of Radiology. He told me that he and his staff had been fascinated by the way I had been able to tolerate the radiation process. He asked me to chronologically go through what I did each day. My days weren't very exciting, just the usual stuff we all do. I got up, showered, walked to the hospital, and waited my turn on the linear accelerator. When the treatment, which lasted but a few minutes, was over, I would walk back to the hotel. The path to the hotel had a stream to jump over. A beautiful herb garden surrounded several buildings I passed. I learned the names, appearance and spelling of a few new herbs each day.

Along the way, there was a deli where I stopped to buy some lunch to take to my hotel room. I always bought a tiny bottle of Inglenook just enough for two small glasses.

Once home, I would relax, eat a bagel with cream cheese and wash it down with a few sips of wine. The warmth of the wine made me sleepy. I would doze off for a wonderful middle-of-the-day nap, a luxury, that before cancer, I had rarely taken advantage of. Oh, it was fun!

When I got to that part of my story, the Chief of Radiology questioned, "Wait, what did you say? Weren't you told not to drink wine during your protocol?"

"No, no one had ever mentioned it."

He looked at me in disbelief.

Maybe the things we don't know are better for us than the things we do know.

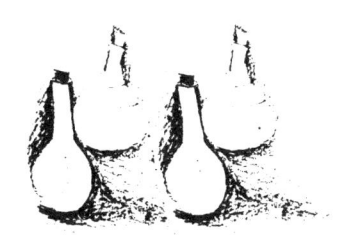

GREEN RUBBER BOOTS

In the house across from us in Akron lived a family of four. The father worked for a large national corporation. They had moved every several years as he was promoted within the company. The mother was a free spirit. She was not tied down to housework, fixing meals or carting children to and from activities.

The children were Gretchen, who was about seven, and Peter, who was four. Peter wandered the neighborhood. We all cared for him and for Gretchen. Peter always wore his high green rubber boots, rain or shine, no matter how hot or cold it was, with no socks and always on the wrong feet. His little head just reached the bottom of the screen in our side door. He ate and visited all over the neighborhood. Dad was always "working" and mom "was playing golf, or getting her hair combed, or colored, or "done".

We grew to love Peter and Gretchen. At seven, Gretchen was a little mother to Peter. She tried to get him to wear his tennis shoes but he wouldn't hear of it. He loved his green rubber boots. He was always ready for a flood.

The fact that I was bald and always wearing a scarf didn't seem to matter to them. They made me feel okay. To them, I wasn't a cancer patient. I was the lady across the street who always had something that was tasty for them to eat and drink. Some afternoons I would get out paints and magic markers. Art time was fun time. We never discussed my health. We laughed and enjoyed our time together.

One day, out of the blue, they arrived at the front door, holding hands. I was a bit surprised since they usually just knocked on the side door or even just came in the unlocked screen door. This day was different. They were as formal as a four and seven year old could be. They were dressed in their good clothes except, of course, for Peter's green rubber boots, on the wrong feet; toes pointing humorously to the outside. I invited them in. They said no, that they couldn't stay. They had just come over to say goodbye.

"Our dad's been transferred. We're moving to South Carolina." Gee, I was sorry. I told them I'd miss their daily visits. And then in all her innocence, Gretchen politely expressed how sorry she was that I was going to die.

"Going to die?" I asked. "Whoever told you that?"

"Oh," she said, "everyone in the neighborhood knows. They're all talking about it. Don't you know you're sick and that you're dying?"

It only takes one innocent question from a child to learn what the latest rumor is in the neighborhood.

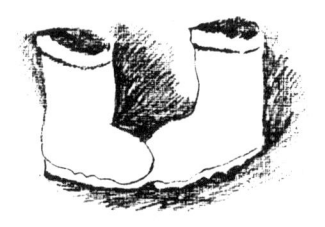

ANNIVERSARY DINNER

Jerry and I were married in 1961. On our 18th anniversary, I was in the midst of my chemotherapy treatments. I wanted our anniversary to be special. It was important to me that for one short evening we set the disease of cancer aside and celebrate those happy, carefree 17 years.

Somehow, getting ready to face the world became more and more difficult as I looked in the mirror each morning. Another day of baldness.

Another day of people asking, "How are you?"

Their faces told me how they thought I was. Another day of my new freedom. I had no drive to Kent State University. I had no classes to teach. I had no students to motivate.

And so, on August 5, 1979, I started early to prepare for that special evening of celebration. Carefully, I selected clothing that would make me feel good about myself.

My high-necked, dark eggplant silk blouse had been a real find, along with a lovely cotton scarf with a design which included the same wonderful color. I decided they were perfect for the evening.

I had discovered someplace along the way that if I secured a Kotex Light Day Pad with its adhesive strip across my head where my hairline once was, I looked as though I had hair under the scarf I had learned to tie behind one ear. Once tied, I also discovered that if I put a piece of wrinkled tissue paper up and under the back of the scarf, it gave the appearance of having my hair in a bun in the back. Well, with Kotex and tissue paper in place and some large gold hoop earrings, out we went to our favorite restaurant for a quiet evening.

The dining room was cozy, the lights were turned down, and there were candles on each table. We were escorted to a nice little table for two. Just around a corner sat a man and woman. I could see the gentleman. The woman was not in my vision. As I approached the table, I held my head high, not wanting the Kotex or the tissue to move from their assigned places.

Just as I sat down, I heard the man I had noticed at the next table say to his wife, "Oh, you should see the exotic woman who just sat down!"

Exotic! Oh, how I needed that! I really never wanted then or now to be thought of as exotic but it did so much for my mood at the time.

It's amazing how soft lighting, candles on the tables, a Light Day Kotex stuck to your head, and a wad of tissue tucked carefully under a scarf can produce an illusion. We see only what is presented to us. Life is not always what it seems to be.

Can you imagine what the reaction of that kind gentleman would have been if my trusty scarf had accidentally fallen off or come untied?

We laughed all the way home. It had, indeed, been an exotic evening.

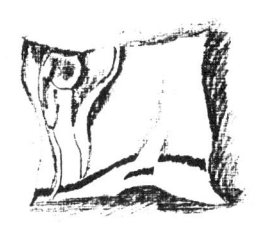

THE CIGARETTE STORY

I smoked a pack of Salem cigarettes a day for 15 years. When we departed for the National Institutes of Health, I packed a carton of "my bad habit" snugly in my suitcase anticipating the fact that there would be no place to buy cigarettes at the hospital. In 1979, smoke-free buildings were unheard of.

We were permitted to smoke in the central lounge areas. One hot, humid evening twenty-some of us in various stages of our disease were clustered together, clad in our nightgowns. I looked around the room. I examined each face. Most were much younger than my 42 years. We were from all parts of the world. What had done this to us, I wondered? I tried to make some sense of it all.

We were all so different; our backgrounds were terribly diverse.

Gradually I realized that we did have commonalities. We had two. One, we all had the same cancer; and two, we were all smoking.

The young man beside me looked like Robert Redford and Paul Newman combined. His bright blue terry cloth robe that matched his beautiful blue eyes hung open. In an earlier surgery one arm had been amputated and now, down his chest were the clamps that told of recent lung surgery. That strong visual image rang an alarm in my brain.

"Why am I smoking this ugly thing?" I asked myself.

That was what it took for me to come to grips with my bad habit. While I had attempted to quit many times before, those attempts usually ended by noon the following day.

That evening I walked to my room, recovered the nearly full carton of Salems I had brought from home and before throwing it into the brown plastic wastebasket in the lounge, I announced to the group, "I'm never smoking another one of these!"

It felt good. I was sure this time. I would never smoke again. Hallelujah!

As I went back to my room to avoid the smoke-filled area, already acting the part of a non-smoker, I watched only to see a very young lady with one leg amputated because of a sarcoma tumor hop over to the wastebasket to retrieve my carton of Salems.

"I can't believe you're throwing these perfectly good cigarettes away!" she exclaimed.

I am as certain today as I was the day I threw away those cigarettes that cigarette smoking causes cancer.

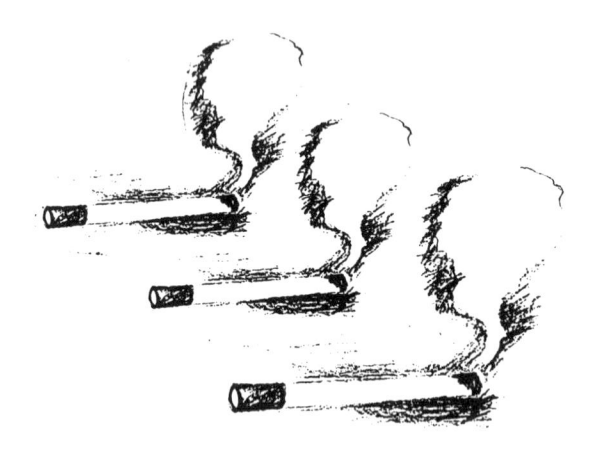

THE ART EXHIBIT

In a course I taught at Kent State University, we used a delightful textbook by Victor Lowenfeld entitled **The Creative and Mental Growth of the Child,** in which Dr. Lowenfeld states that the more senses involved in any learning experience, the more intense the learning. In my classes, I would include activities that would enhance a variety of learning behaviors. In creating sounds and smells, tastes and a variety of feeling sensations, learning experiences were intensified. The smell of freshly baked bread combined with the taste of homemade strawberry jam motivated students to draw themselves in greater detail. Their self portraits included opened mouths with teeth dripping with the red sticky jam, hands holding the bread, their eyes all aglow as they devoured their tasty treat.

This part of a course in creativity excited me. I had proof that it worked. It was true, the more senses involved in an experience the stronger the experience. This was a belief I had related only to art education. I had never given it much thought concerning other areas of life.

Chemotherapy intensified my sense of smell. As the chemotherapy made its way through my body, it would burn the inside of my nose as it slowly inched its way through my system. When I reported for radiation each morning, I could actually smell the people in the room who were taking the same drugs that I was taking. Today, I am overly sensitive to various odors especially perfumes of all kinds. Department stores are difficult for me to tolerate because of their centralized cosmetic areas.

The Adriamycin was bright red in color. When I saw bright red I could actually smell the smells of the drugs. The overlapping of my senses, the interaction of smells and sounds with colors and textures has heightened my perceptions. Since having cancer, my own art work has been impacted by these changes in my perceptual awareness.

Several years after being well, I was asked by a local gallery owner to have a retrospective show of my paintings. It was exciting to gather and assemble work done over a period of some thirty years. The gallery curator hung the work in chronological order. The evening of the opening, it was an amazing awakening for me to see how my work had changed after my cancer experience. I hadn't really realized it prior to the show. There was an invisible line that seemed to separate my work into two very distinct groups. There was what I call a BC group and an AC group. Before cancer, the colors were clean and clear but subtle and sometimes drab. The pieces were smaller and more timid. I had obviously taken fewer risks. There seemed to be a heavy emphasis on the visual.

After cancer my work included big, bold detailed, sure statements about my world and how I perceived it. Colors moved; they "made sounds" as they clearly spoke to the viewers.

People who attended the opening were fascinated by that invisible line. They were able to see the differences. They delighted in realizing that they were able to better understand art and how much of the artist exists in each of his or her visual statements.

My work has stayed very lively. My senses pick up details never evoked before having had cancer. There is less emphasis on the visual impact. Feelings and internal relationships are evidenced.

Subject matter revolves around the simple everyday wonders of life. Electric colors vibrate from the surface of the canvasses. My world seems easier to digest. The beauty of the simple becomes clearer as I paint what surrounds me.

We must be careful to realize some of the good things cancer can do for us. While that may sound like an oxymoron, for me, it is the truth. Today, my senses overlap; they devour my world in a far more unique way than before I experienced the disease of cancer.

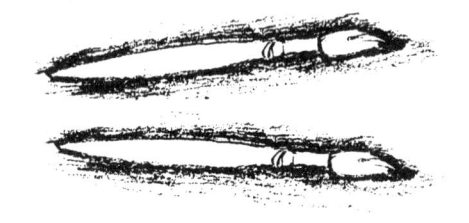

THE PERFECT MOUSE

At one point, I had a National Institutes of Health nurse for a roommate. Her name was Cathy. She was such fun! At night we would sign off 10E, the surgery floor, and wander around the hospital. We would visit the small chapel our Irish chaplain had meticulously created for us. In the quiet of the night, the candle in its red glass holder glowed warmly. It signaled that the Blessed Sacrament was in the small golden tabernacle. Two little, maroon velvet kneelers awaited our knees. We said our little prayers of hope and thanks. The loving Jesuit priest left the key to his office under the gold cover

over the tabernacle so that we could use the 800 line on his telephone. We enjoyed this luxury.

Prowling the research corridors was exciting. My roommate knew her way around the ten story building. One evening while we were in one of the elevators with two men, we overheard their conversation.

One said, "I can't believe he let that perfect specimen get away from him."

"Neither can I," answered his friend. "It seems to be the way he does everything. You find him a special, perfect specimen and he doesn't follow up on it."

Cathy and I glanced at one another. What or who was the perfect specimen? We wondered if their friend had lost the opportunity to meet a young lady they had found for him.

As the elevator neared the eighth floor and they proceeded to exit, we heard, "However could he have let such a perfect mouse go to someone else?"

The scientists are persons unto themselves. They work alone in the middle of the night. They become absorbed in their work, often in tiny spaces, doing what most of us have absolutely no understanding. Whatever would we do without them, and whatever would we do without those perfect mice? They both save lives.

THE ICE CREAM PARLOR

Our days seemed to go quickly. They were filled with radiation treatments, tests, doctor appointments and scans. It was the evenings that seemed to drag on and on. There were five or six of us who wandered around together. We discovered an ice cream parlor that had real home-made ice cream about three blocks down Wisconsin Avenue. If we all had a pretty good day, we would venture out after dinner for some ice cream. People were out and about, walking around in the hot, humid Washington weather.

The first time we arrived at what was to become our favorite place in town, it was packed. Every table was taken. We wondered where we would sit once we had selected our ice cream treats. Involved in our ice cream treat decision, we waited at the counter for our delicious orders. Once they were completed, the servers handed each of us what we had ordered. Hot fudge, pecans, bananas on chocolate ice cream with chocolate sauce. We all had our favorites. As we turned, all wondering where we'd find a table for the five or six of us, we suddenly realized that while we were busy ordering our ice cream, people had quickly finished and left. We almost had the ice cream parlor to ourselves. A few poor souls decided to stay and stare at us. They were probably tourists and didn't know about the government research hospital up the street. It was a strange feeling to be treated so differently from the way I had been treated before cancer. That night we didn't discuss what had happened.

Several nights later Joe announced, "Let's go down to the ice cream parlor and scare all the people away."

Off we went, laughing all the way!

COON DOG MAN

Clarence came from the rolling hills of Kentucky. When he told of his home, his words painted pictures of the green, beautiful place he loved. While Clarence had never learned to read or write, he was perceptive, bright and humorous. Stories of his beloved coon dog entertained us. How he looked forward to his days of going home again! His coon dog was the light of his life and he was sure it anxiously awaited his return.

His home was back and away from the road "where houses should always be built". It was small but contained all the necessities. Clarence took joy in his accomplishments and pride in having never missed a day of work. He was quick to tell of the wonders of his newly-purchased red pick-up truck.

"Wanted one all my life," he proudly proclaimed.

Midway into his treatment, Clarence was permitted to go home for a weekend visit. His caregivers could see his noticeable homesickness. He longed to see his home, his pick-up truck, and most of all, his coon dog. Seldom did he ever mention his wife.

We all wished Clarence goodbye as he joyfully headed home for his long weekend. We were excited for him and we knew he'd return filled with stories of happenings in those green-covered Kentucky hills. He would report on the ventures in his red truck, the warmth of his little hand-built house, and the greeting from his faithful coon dog. The following Sunday morning, five or six of us gathered to eat a little lunch. Eating was not always easy or fun during chemotherapy. Bob, another cancer patient, announced that Clarence was back from his weekend home.

"Back so soon?" we all chimed in.

He wasn't due back until Monday afternoon.

We looked up and saw Clarence come into the dining room with its paper place mats and plastic hanging plants. His face was long. He was filled with gloom. He walked slowly and was a bit bent over, touching each chair for support as he headed in our direction. We all worried Clarence might have had a setback in his treatment, or traveling might have been too much for him.

He slumped into the green plastic circular booth where we were gathered. The heaviness of his heart was contagious. Something terrible had happened. Something awful was wrong. Would he get the courage to share his sadness? Slumped in the booth, surrounded by his new friends, he reported that upon his arrival home, he discovered his wife had sold the house, his red pick-up truck, and had given away his coon dog.

The sadness that accompanies the illness of cancer is often not from the disease itself but from the reactions of the world. Within time, Clarence recovered from his losses, but he never fully returned to being the person that he had been. He did learn, however, that the things we don't know about cancer, the subsequent circumstances, can be more horrible than the disease itself.

We all grew because of Clarence. He showed us that his struggle to be well again was more important than the possessions he had loved so dearly. He could build another home and buy another pick-up truck. We all agreed his coon dog could never be replaced. It would have to become a loving memory.

What fun we had that summer as we watched Clarence learn to read and write!

He would go home a new person.

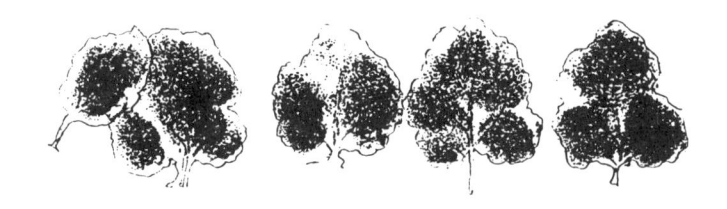

BUDWEISER MAN

Ten days after his first treatment, his hair, like all of ours, fell out. His head was as bald and shiny as all of ours were. Dealing with baldness was not easy for any of us. We tried to laugh about it, but it wasn't easy. Our television sets, the staring of strangers, and the sad eyes of those who loved us, told us that ours was a sorry plight. No more brushing, washing, conditioning, curling, cutting, perming, ratting, teasing, fluffing, coloring, streaking, or even having a "bad hair day" for us! Our bald heads reminded us every morning as we looked in the mirror that we were ill. They told us our baldness was proof the chemotherapy was working. Hair cells like cancer cells are fast growing. Signs reading "God created only a few perfect heads, the rest he covered with hair" were hung in various places to make us laugh at our predicament. We tried not to let the staring of strangers or the television commercials filled with hair products, bother us.

Our **Budweiser Man** solved his bald head problem by using his loved, old friend, his Budweiser hat. He was never without this badly worn hat which told of his favorite drink. The old hat was now there to help and comfort him when he needed it most.

He told us that at one time he had almost thrown it away. But, without knowing why, he had decided to keep "his old friend". Little did he realize then how much he would need that hat. He never took it off. It became part of him. I guess his is a story that tells us that sometimes something unimportant in health can become very important during illness. Cancer taps our creativity and our resources. It stretches us to see new meaning in the simplest of things.

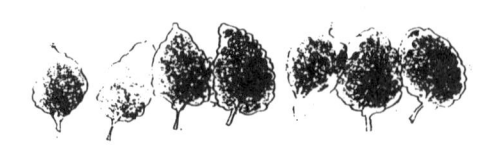

NOT THE MEASLES OR MUMPS

Illness before cancer is fairly predictable. We have known stages since childhood. Early signs start — a headache, a sore throat, a fever, indigestion, diarrhea. We know something is wrong. A trip to the drug store usually follows. A talk with the pharmacist, an over the counter medication, rest, lots of fluids and in several days it's over, gone. If things stay the same or get worse, it's off to the family doctor. He or she writes a secret message in some sort of "doctor writing code" on a little white prescription pad, signs his or her name as some unique scribble his or her third grade teacher would frown upon and tells us to rest and eat chicken noodle soup. In a week to ten days, it's gone. We are annoyed that we had to step off the escalator of life for such a long time and we are sure the world just can't get along without us. In fact, it's become fashionable to go to work in spite of the illness and tell everyone how terrible we feel. Thus, others can have what we have and it will go around and around the work place. If all goes as predicted, we might even get it back.

The process is about the same with the measles, we get red spots; with mumps, we get lumps; with a cold, we get a stuffy nose. We have known all of them. And, in the "instant" society we have created we know that it will go away sooner or later. After all, the world needs us. We are important. There is no time to be sick. Sick is what happens to other people. Sick is for old people. We are never going to be old or sick.

Finding out you have cancer is different. The process is dramatically different. There is no trip to the drug store, no over the counter drugs, no one-time prescription, no rash, no stuffy nose, and chicken soup just won't cut it; nor, will a week of bed rest. It's there, every morning, every afternoon, every night.

The world continues. Friends try to be supportive. The road to wellness begins. It's long. It can be sad, annoying. Time marches on. Digesting the diagnosis isn't easy.

Swallowing is difficult. There's an invisible lump in your throat and a flutter in your stomach. Your mind never stops. All of life zooms through your brain. Happy things linger. The time you spent doing unimportant things seems silly and wasted. The future is a blur. You rehearse for a variety of events. Each day the "what if's" loom over you.

Medical people say things like "get your life in order." I remember spending days trying to figure out just exactly what that meant. I found myself cleaning out my desk drawers and sorting through clothing. It was difficult to part with things that held happy memories. There seemed to be a need to put things in proper places. I threw away stubby pencils, sharpened others. I tested the small box of ball point pens in the drawer beside the telephone book. I threw away the ones that wouldn't work on the first try. Magic Markers that had lost their strength were pitched.

Our Christmas things bothered me. Had I put them away neatly? Would someone else be able to find things easily? Each year since that fateful time, I carefully tuck Christmas decorations away making sure each is wrapped and labeled. I say goodbye to some of my favorite things. I hopefully want to see them again the next year.

I wrote notes and letters to people I loved and to some I hadn't seen in years. I needed to tell people how good they had been to me, that I liked them very much and that I remembered some significant, fun times we had had together.

I wrote long, detailed instructions for my funeral. I wanted to be buried in a white flannel nightgown with warm slippers on my feet. The funeral director had asked me to remember my mother's panty hose when I assembled her things after she had died. I didn't want to wear those uncomfortable, tight ugly things to Heaven. I planned the music selections. I wanted people to be happy. I wanted them to celebrate life.

It was all very confusing. Trying to understand why the chemotherapy made me sicker than when I started was difficult. It's like going backwards in order to move forward. Contradictions abound. Nothing seems predictable. Reality finally surfaces. Days linger. More of the same each month. Rigid routines are set in place; a blood test every Friday morning, holes poked in each arm. Taking part in life gets harder and harder. People ask questions. People tell one sad cancer story after the other. I have heard them all. Details of the people they knew who had died of cancer. "Aunt Sally's mastectomy disfigured her. It came back anyhow. Gone in six months." "I know how you feel" becomes a haunting over-repeated message. Being polite, being a patient listener gets harder and harder.

One day when I was in a nice little greeting card shop, I overheard a shopper ask the owner of the shop if she had any cards for cancer patients. Innocently, I pointed to where the get well cards were.

She replied, "No, Honey, I need a card for a cancer patient. A get well card wouldn't be appropriate."

We weren't getting better in the eyes of many. We could tell what they were thinking. Shortly after that time, I noticed that the card companies started making their "Cope Lines", cards with messages like "Hang in there", "Tomorrow will be brighter", or "In spite of it all, we love you." It was easy to see this wasn't just any illness. Its unpredictable behavior was misunderstood. It is, indeed, a frightening disease. To many, it equates death. It doesn't take long to realize that cancer isn't the measles or the mumps!

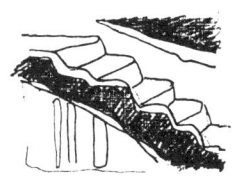

THE HOTEL IS FULL

For subsequent follow up visits, we were responsible to make our own hotel reservations. NIH provided a list of hotels, telephone numbers and room rates. We were careful to call in plenty of time.

Looking forward to one of my visits, I called a hotel on Pooks Hill. I was connected with the lady in charge of reservations.

Cheerfully, I announced in reply to her request to help me, "Yes, I am a cancer patient coming to Bethesda for my NIH appointment." I added the days I needed a room.

"Oh," she said, after an acceptable amount of time, "I'm afraid the hotel is full at that time. Sorry."

I put down the receiver in disappointment. How could the hotel be full this far from the days I requested? Where else should I call? That voice stayed with me. "Sorry, we're full."

After contemplating the telephone experience, I decided to try again. This time I re-worded my introduction.

"Hello, I am Dr. Kathleen Whitmer coming to Bethesda for a conference at NIH."

Again, I gave her the dates for which I'd need a room.

Whether it was to my surprise or not, I am not sure, for she quickly replied, "Oh, yes, Dr. Whitmer, we have a lovely room," and then as if that were not enough she added "and we have a nice discounted package for you."

No room in the inn for the cancer patient. A room with a view at a special rate for the healthy doctor.

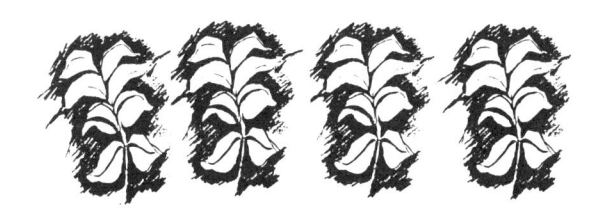

TAXI CAB RIDE

It was fall in DC. The trees were in full color. Warm wool sweaters were back from their summer hibernation. My flight into Washington National Airport was uneventful. I had learned to ask for a window seat. It was fun to search for the NIH buildings as we neared the Washington area. I had certain landmarks that identified directions and areas. The Pentagon with its neatly measured five even sides was just like Sister Bridgette said it was when I was in the fifth grade. Circles of streets radiating into neighborhoods brought back memories of a course in perspective I had taken in college. We learned the various ways cities were planned. Washington had been planned in a "wagon wheel" concept, a circle with streets radiating from that circle. Dupont Circle became a favorite area of mine. The Folk Art Museum filled long afternoons as did the Phillips Museum.

In the fall of 1985, now six years cancer-free, I spent three days having tests and doctor appointments. Both proved me well for one more year. I had grown to love all that my visits included: the smell of the air, the cobblestone drive that led to the main entrance of the Clinical Center, the always predictable procedures and the warm welcomes.

I was elated that things were perfectly fine. My cancer had not returned. I was well. It's a hard feeling to describe to people who have never experienced the disease of cancer. People generally try hard to identify with one another.

"Oh, I know just how you feel," they often tell one another.

Why do we do that? We clearly know from all of life's experiences that we just cannot know how something feels to someone else unless we have felt it ourselves. And even then, individual circumstances can change each experience.

That fall afternoon, with another good report under my belt, I headed for the transportation area. It was time to get a flight home. I wore the Irish cream wool cardigan sweater Aunt Mary had brought back to me from her trip to Ireland. The weather was perfect for it.

The travel department found a flight leaving National Airport for Cleveland. I'd have to rush if I were to make it. The Director of Transportation said he would call a cab rather than have me wait for the shuttle. There wasn't time for that. I hated to see such an expense. A cab for just one person seemed excessive.

I was assured not to worry. There was another lady who needed to get to the airport quickly for her flight. We could share the same taxi. That sounded fine to me. I stood under the protective portico awaiting the taxi.

A nice little lady walked slowly from the building to where I was standing. The cab arrived. Mother had taught us that in such cases it was polite to get in first so that the other person need not slide across the seat to the other side. I slid in, across the worn, cracked leather-like taxi seat. The small lady followed me. The driver slammed the door.

As we inched our way from the ten story building, I glanced out the rear window. I liked finding "my floor" and mentally saying goodbye. I had grown to appreciate all this place meant to me. It had been good to me.

My new friend and I both had on Irish wool sweaters. Hers had a belt with two leather buttons to match the row of buttons that marched neatly down its front. She sat peacefully. After one last look at the Clinical Center, I settled in for the forty-five minute ride to the airport.

Just as I looked away from the building, I announced, "I'd give my right arm to live close enough to this place so that I could volunteer every day. What a wonderful place it is!"

She looked straight into my eyes, her kind face receptive to my being with her.

In response to my statement she replied, "Let's not discuss right arms. This is the first time I've been out without mine. I'm leaving it behind. I had it amputated a month ago because of a sarcoma tumor."

The empty right sleeve of her creamy Irish wool sweater was tucked neatly into her pocket. One folded hand rested on her lap. My body froze and then I got hot. My breath shortened.

How could I have said such a terrible thing? Horrified, I tried to apologize. Graciously, she dismissed my stupidity.

"I'll have to get used to such statements sooner or later. Please don't feel bad."

The ride to the airport was quiet. I chastised myself then, and even telling the story all these years later makes me a little sick. I have tried to learn to think before I speak. Today when I hear people foolishly say, "Oh, I'd die for a coat like that," or "It's to die for," or "I'd kill to have a car like that," I realize over again what really silly and untrue statements can come out of our silly mouths!

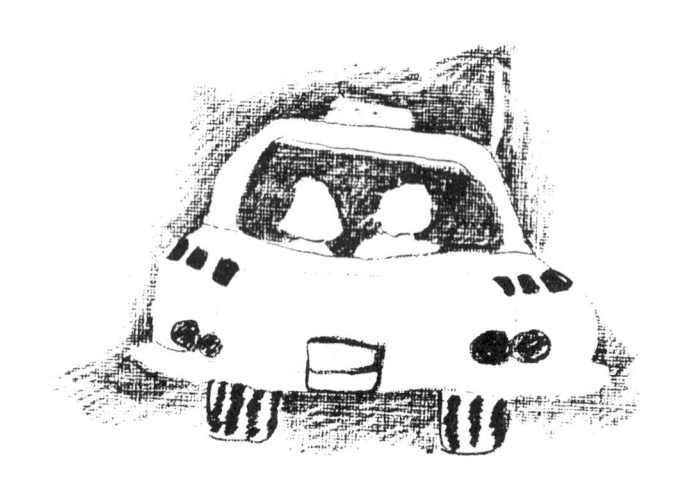

THE FIRST MRS. WHITMER

A little over a year after I returned home from my chemotherapy treatments, I was asked by a local woman's civic organization to sit in on one of its meetings. They wanted help with their plans for a fund raiser. With my art background, I could help them with ideas about colors, invitations and creative approaches to attracting interest in their venture.

While straight salt and pepper gray hair had fallen out, I had a beautiful new head of black curly hair. The year of baldness had had its rewards. I wore a simple white blouse and a blue skirt with a wide wallpaper-like deep border around the bottom. Years ago, Aunt Mary had given me a lovely old, deep blue lapis ring that had been Aunt Mame's. I wore it almost every day since the day that she had given it to me.

I didn't know the women in the group personally. One lady looked vaguely familiar. I noticed that she was staring at me. She examined me carefully.

Every now and then I caught her glance. She seemed puzzled. I felt a little uncomfortable. I checked to see if I had forgotten anything or if I had accidentally put on mismatched shoes. I decided that she liked the blue bordered skirt. Others had.

The meeting was run efficiently by the president of the organization. Light refreshments were served after the meeting was adjourned. The ladies cheerfully mingled. Within moments, the lady who had been carefully examining me was at my side. She held a china tea cup in her well-manicured hands. She looked into my face and stated that she had been looking at me and had been trying to figure out something. She needn't have told me; I had felt her scrutiny.

And, in a loud and clear voice she asked, "Do you own an Irish setter?"

I replied positively.

And then she asked, "Well, are you the first Mrs. Whitmer?"

She seemed puzzled.

Was I the first Mrs. Whitmer? I was confused. Well, yes and no, Jerry's mother was a Mrs. Whitmer. His brothers' wives were all Mrs. Whitmers. Was I the first Mrs. Whitmer?

I responded, "Yes, I am the first Mrs. Jerry Whitmer."

Wide-eyed and finally satisfied with the answer, she removed one hand from her blue teacup, slapped her thigh as she announced as plain as day, "Lord, I heard you died. I've been sitting here all afternoon wondering how that man found a second wife that looked so much like his first wife. Except for the black curly hair, you look exactly like you did the evening we met on the corner of Peach Road and Firsthaven one warm summer evening years ago. You and your husband were walking your Irish setter. I especially remember that lovely old blue lapis ring."

She had decided that I was a new wife, the second Mrs. Whitmer sporting a better head of hair than the first and wearing the jewelry of the first. How bad news travels. Why hadn't the good news of my recovery traveled as fast?

When I got home the events of the day wouldn't leave me. Would there ever be a second Mrs. Whitmer? Who knows? There are things we can control and there are things we will never control. That there could be a second Mrs. Whitmer some day was not for me to say. Who knows the future? Who wants to know it?

When my husband came in from work that evening, he found me writing on a yellow legal pad. I had drawn a line vertically down the middle of the top page. I had gone to my jewelry drawer and had carefully listed each piece of jewelry: Grandma Minnie's bracelet given to her on her 16th birthday, my wedding pearls, Aunt Mame's diamond broach, cousin John's triple gold Tiffany 1929 signature ring, and some lovely things that Jerry had bought me over the years. The list wasn't long but it included some old things filled with history and memories. I then listed my favorite friends and relatives in the second column. I matched the person with the piece of jewelry I thought best suited each.

Yes, it was true. I really could not determine the future. I knew not whether there would be a second Mrs. Whitmer. I could, however, control the fact that she would have to wear her own jewelry, not mine.

At first, realizing people had discussed my death startled me. Then I became more realistic. People talk about people and in a world where the media, newspapers, and television dwell entirely on the negative, it is easy for us to fall into the same pattern. People pass along information, adding, changing, eliminating, editing as they see fit; each giving it his or her own flair.

I decided that I could have easily cried about this sad fact or I could accept it as part of what makes us all human. And being human is not always being perfect.

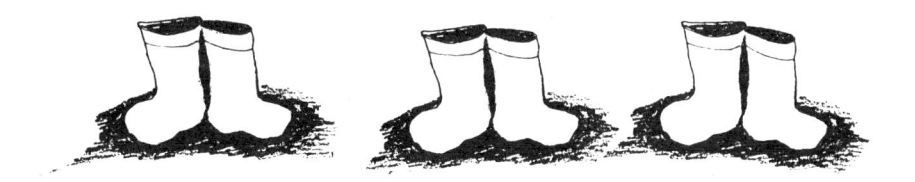

CANCER LADY

Years after having had cancer, I continue to work with cancer patients. My work brings me great joy. I found that when I was sick and going through the process of getting well, it was hard to be both the patient and the advocate. All my energy had to go into the concentration it takes to focus on wellness. The battles about cancer and its insurmountable side issues had to be someone else's problem.

Today I search for answers for patients too exhausted to do their own research. I help to listen as their caregivers give them instructions. I accompany them to their radiation appointments. We carefully go over their diets together. I always share with them the kinds of foods that others found nutritious and tolerable.

It has become easier and easier for me to give my cancer friends the hope that I longed for all those years ago. With love and admiration, I sit by their bedsides as they undergo the drudgery of the chemicals they must take to kill those "out of control adolescent" cancer cells. The families of the cancer patients suffer greatly. They feel such a struggle within and want so badly to be able to make the cancer go away.

My work is not hard. It is not, because cancer patients have a remarkable spirit. They are uplifting, cheerful, giving, and always filled with gratitude. And they respond positively to the smallest piece of helpful information.

One day not long ago, after a day on the oncology floor at a local hospital, I stopped at the grocery store for a few fresh things for our night's dinner. As I reached for a bundle of asparagus, from across the store I heard one shopper exclaim to another "Oh look, there is the "cancer lady". Since they were looking in my direction, I glanced over my shoulder to see about whom they were talking.

Much to my surprise, all that was over my shoulder was the fresh vegetable case. That "cancer lady" whom they recognized was I. For a moment I stood confused. The "cancer lady"? What a strange title. When had that come to be? And then, I realized that while others might shun even the notion of such a title, I felt a sort of satisfaction that comes only from such a rare and unusual happening. I left the grocery store, my asparagus tucked into the brown bag along with a few other goodies. Surviving cancer can give you a title more exciting than king, queen, movie star, or sports hero.

That day, I came to the conclusion that having an experience with cancer and not telling about it, keeping it a secret and denying it, and hoping no one would know, would have really been wrong for me.

The truth of the good and the bad in our lives gives others hope and gives a purpose to being human. We begin our lives with dreams and goals and hope our preparation will lead us to happiness and success. At times, we are forced to wander from our usual expected paths. The ability to remain flexible and positive in spite of the rough path can in itself be more satisfying than traveling a smooth, predictable journey.

LOTS OF LASTS

Cancer is like a car being stolen or a house being broken into; alarms go off. The alarm signal is so loud you need to cover your ears. When I heard the words, I couldn't remember any sounds that followed. Something had sneaked into my body and had started to destroy it from within. It was robbing my blood system of healthy cells. I was driving down the street with my health in the back seat. Stop! Call for help! Don't let it happen. It's mine. I need it to live. I wanted things to be like they had always been.

We adjust to having a car stolen and to having things robbed from our homes. Adjusting to the diagnosis of cancer isn't as easy. I couldn't go out and buy new blood cells, nor could I say, "Oh, well, I never needed all those things anyhow."

Our bodies, once perfect, symmetrically designed machines, are disfigured. Mine was sliced down the right side. Bulletin board-like staples called clamps held the slice together. When the bandages were removed for the first time, all I could say about the disfigurement was, "Oh, my!" Then I counted how many staples there were. How long would they be there? How were they going to be removed?

Beside the neat row of metal staples was a rubber tube stuck inside a little hole in my flesh. It had a large silver safety pin on the end closest to my skin so that it would not disappear into the hole. It reminded me of quicksand. It was there to drain the sliced pancreas. It was removed several days after surgery. It left a tiny scar as a reminder.

The slice healed. A seam now remains where it was. I had never had a need to wear a bikini. Now, I would never wear one for sure.

For the second surgery to remove any new growth, the NIH surgeon decided to reopen the original incision. It was back to the original spot. It had just healed. More clamps. The morning the Chief of Surgery uncovered the newly clamped slice, I watched his face. He seemed not to like what he saw. I looked down cautiously. The slice now had a pleat in it. Damn!

A group of interns huddled around their teacher. Their eyes told of a slight error.

"Who closed?" the master surgeon gruffly asked.

"Smith," they all chimed.

I don't know where Smith is today but I do know that I have a pucker along my waist line that I don't like. It's no big thing. I've just had to learn to buy clothing a bit larger because the pucker doesn't like to be pinched.

Once I was home recuperating, I felt as though someone else's body hung from my neck. Most of my favorite clothes felt wrong. It took longer to do everything. I got up later in the morning and needed to go to bed earlier each evening. People seemed to act differently. Telephone calls were guarded. The grocery store seemed larger. Spaces of time changed. Afternoons were long while mornings were short. The need to stay in harmony was all-consuming. I had to work at it.

Later, I was to find that my right leg was affected by the radiation. Because it's just a tad shorter, I have a backache now and then. The right side of my body is smaller.

Radiation shrunk the symmetrical machine. Then, heart problems started to cause limitations. A navy blue handicapped sticker now hangs from the car mirror. Handicapped parking is appreciated.

Soon I realized it helped if I focused on the positives of the disabilities. I can no longer carry groceries from the car to the kitchen. I can no longer iron. The basement is almost off limits. Rest comes easily. People understand. I have become selective about saying "Yes."

After cancer, a sort of discrimination sneaks into our lives. When I was bald, there was a shower given by an important lady in town for a good friend's daughter. My covered bald head might have spoiled the happiness of the day, so I wasn't to be invited. I learned of the happening by accident. It made me sad. While I was a little different on the outside, I was the same person on the inside. Discrimination takes on all forms. It can be very subtle. You know it one way or another. It hurts.

The shuttle trips we took as patients into DC to visit spots of interest brought stares and whispers.

"What do you suppose is wrong with those people?" friends asked one another as we exited the bus.

They covered their mouths with their hands. They tried to be careful not to be overheard. Anyplace there was a line of people waiting their turn, we were encouraged to go to the front of the line. They looked at us as though, if we didn't go to the front of the line, we'd never stay alive long enough to see whatever it was we were there to see.

Uncomfortable feelings become omnipresent. A constant wonderment of feelings is strangely different. The need to rid myself of the new, uncomfortable feelings grew great. Comfort came from prayer and from the realization that I was in charge of those feelings. Thoughts always precede feelings. How I thought affected how I felt. I had to stop what I was doing when uncomfortable feelings began and I had to change my "think tape". Happy thoughts produce happy feelings.

For me, death had always been a part of the process of living, but it had never been so predictable or clearly set. The mystery of the unknown kept moving. The "last" of things started to take shape. This might be my "last" birthday. This Christmas might be our "last" Christmas. More pictures were taken. People worked hard to make events especially nice. There might not be others.

And now 18 years later, there have been 18 more birthdays, 18 more Christmases, 18 more winters and summers. There have been lots of "lasts"! Lasts do accumulate before you know it!

THE DOCTORS AFTER CANCER

Before cancer, I had one doctor. I saw him once a year whether I needed to or not. It seemed like the right thing to do.

Let me tell you what happens after cancer. With the diagnosis comes a surgeon, followed by a radiologist and an oncologist. The surgeon "opens" and "closes".

He or she usually says, "Well, I think we got it all."

After he or she leaves the room, you lie back, glad it's all over and you decide that within weeks life will be back to normal.

The doctors' words haunt you. "I think we got it all," repeats itself. "Think" seems to say "well, maybe." "We" suggests the surgeon wasn't the only person in on the project and "it" means he or she can't stand saying the word cancer, let alone saying it to another person. Doctors hate cancer as much as we do. They are as human as we are.

The oncologist works on the battlefield. He has seen the casualties. He talks of chemicals that are going to be used to fight the bad cells. The chemicals have names as long as your arm and are impossible to spell. Several minutes into the conversation you lose track of the what's and the when's. Weeks of therapy are explained.

I found myself wanting to yell out, "Wait! Just tell me about this week."

When the oncologist asks if you have any questions, there are none. At night, at home, alone in bed, questions flood your mind. When? Why? How? Where? How long? Was it 80% or 60%? Would my hair fall out all at once or a little at a time? Convinced that the process will never end, sleep is difficult.

The radiologist speaks in another tongue. Beams, rays, linear radiation goes to the "spot". Like a spot on a dog, you think. It will eradicate that "spot". "It will also kill everything in its path." In my case, my right kidney was unfortunate enough to be in the path of the radiation. Gone. Zapped. Never to show on an examination again.

During the first nuclear medicine test after the completion of radiation, the technician asked, "Where's your right kidney? I can't seem to find it."

How was I supposed to know where it was? I never saw it go anywhere. Zapped! Gone!

Now a "kidney man" was called in along with a specialist to examine my esophagus. The endoscopy showed stomach problems and a hiatal hernia. The neurologist came next. Neuropathy was caused by the chemicals. Numb feet and numb fingers became everyday occurences; warm socks and gloves became necessities.

The dreaded "colon man" does his yearly colondoscopies. He allows me to rest on my side and look at a television screen where I can watch the instrument travel up the beautiful red abstract streets of my intestine. Fascinating. A former student from my junior high school teaching days helps to administer the embarrassing procedure.

"Everything will be fine, Mrs. Whitmer," she assures me.

Yesterday, she was only a child of twelve, a sweet seventh grader. As teachers, we never think our students will see us years later in such helpless situations.

Finally, as things started to smooth out for me, it became hard to walk up steps. I was short of breath. In came the cardiologist. CHF. Letters that spelled out heart problems. The experimental chemotherapy was toxic. The left ventricle of the heart decided to grow big and work half the time. It was tired of the assault it had had. Heart medicine caused problems that called for more specialists. Arrhythmia, irregular heart beats, brought with it medicine that, along with a variety of pretty scary side effects, can turn you blue.

"Even the whites of your eyes," I was told.

Each morning I looked to see if I had turned blue. It never happened. However, the rim of my brown eyes did turn blue. That brought with it trips to the opthalmologist.

Because heart medicine can be hard on mouth tissue, dental examinations were moved from once a year to every three months. The gynecologist decided I became a "high risk" patient so his appointments were scheduled for every three months also.

This started out as a short little story to warn some and make others laugh. It's made me laugh. Doctor, doctors, doctors! I could write another book just about them.

I have learned they hate lists of questions prepared prior to a visit. Generally, they like you to be quiet, speak when spoken to; and it's a rare one who sits down, relaxes and tells you about his dog's bad haircut or his kid's soccer game he coached the night before. As brilliant young people, they are hard-working, loving human beings who are misunderstood. They worked years to make their parents proud. They have to learn to accept criticism, receive little praise and be constantly reminded by the unsympathetic public that they make too much money and play too much golf, neither of which is true. They are blamed for making people wait much too long and for having outdated magazines in their waiting rooms. Their careers are short, their hours are long; yet their spirits remain high. They are a breed all their own. Whatever would we do without them?

I have learned to take a good book to any appointment along with the ears and the heart of another person. It's difficult to be the patient and the advocate at the same time. I have found that knowing lots of doctors has some real advantages. High on the list is life.

Cancer left me with a list of side effects. It would be unfair of me to suggest that surviving cancer means walking away carefree and feeling like a twenty year old. It has, however, given me the joy of all the things included in being a survivor of any tragedy.

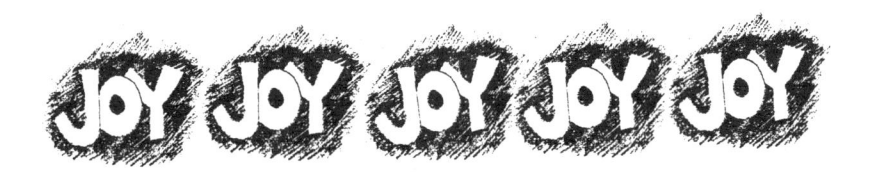

JOY JOY JOY JOY JOY

RETIREMENT

We are working people. We are closely tied to what we do. We frequently are introduced by name followed by our line of work. I had always been, Mrs. Whitmer, Art Professor. Cancer changed that. Perhaps I was to blame. I could not hide or remain silent about my illness. Even when a well-meaning physician recommended that I "get on with life", I found I needed to be verbal and honest, hopeful and optimistic. My doctors recommended that I retire from my career as an art professor due to the damage the experimental chemotherapy had done to my heart. It was not easy. I identified with my work. It was who I was. I knew little else. My job filled my waking hours. In one short week I went from Kathleen Whitmer, Art Professor, to Kathleen Whitmer, Cancer Patient. It was as though one identity was replaced by another. It took time to adjust to the change.

In arranging for my disability retirement, I had to work through the Ohio Teachers Retirement Program at the University. A nice lady in that office worked hard trying to understand how this was all to fall into place. She seemed confused by the process. I had had sick days that had accumulated and when I had used all of them, the retirement plan was to go into effect. One afternoon as we talked through the plan, I sensed her frustration. I apologized for causing her what seemed to be unusual problems. She was flustered. She was unable to comprehend what was to happen.

In response to my apology for causing her what seemed like unsolvable problems, she replied, "Well, Mrs. Whitmer, I'm confused because I've never had a person live as long as you have with your illness. I don't know what the procedure is."

Retirement brings with it a new sense of self, a new sense of time, a new sense of worth and a new sense of identity. It also helps if it brings with it a good sense of humor.

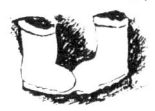

NOTHING HAS TO GO RIGHT

All along the way, I became more and more aware of the meaning of happiness. Since childhood I have been fascinated by the notion of happiness. Why was Sister Gemma so much happier than Sister Marie? Why did I learn more from Sister Gemma even though she taught me a much harder subject?

As a teacher, I wondered why some students were exceptionally content and happy while others were miserable most of the time. Why did some teachers hate Monday morning? Why were they always wishing for Friday afternoon while some couldn't wait for the next class period to begin?

I find myself examining people in the checkout line in the grocery store and people riding in cars stopped at traffic lights beside me. Why are some of these people happy and animated while others are grumpy and even mean-looking?

While I agree that there are degrees of happiness, I continue to wonder just what is in the making of a happy person?

We live in a society where we are bombarded with information. We have Geraldo, Sally Jessie, and Oprah with their panels of "experts" feeding us information; yet we long for knowledge.

We have a constant array of mixed messages. One message says eat chicken, while another says don't eat chicken. We're told to eat vegetables, yet we're told vegetables have been sprayed with chemicals and waxed. The 80's told us we had to run and jump, skip and jog. The 90's added weight lifting, boxing and personal trainers to the list. And now, the all perfect "abs" are a must.

We're told not to eat red meat because of the hormones, but told to take hormones if we want to stay young. We are flooded with talk of heterosexuals, bisexuals, homosexuals, sexual identity, sex changes, sexual freedom, the sexual revolution, sexual harassment and even sexually correct language. Some of us grew up when the word sex was just a three letter word.

If we're too fat, we're told to take a pill. If we don't want a baby, we're told to take a pill. If we're constipated, we're told to take a pill. We're told to take an aspirin every day. We have Mylanta I and Mylanta II. We have low cholesterol and high cholesterol, good cholesterol and bad cholesterol.

There's low salt and no salt. People with curly hair get it straightened, while people with straight hair get it curled. Gray haired women are old, while gray haired men are distinguished.

We have instant orange juice, instant coffee, instant potatoes and fast food. Yes, we have mixed messages in this mixed-up world of ours. How are we to be happy? Is it possible?

Can you remember when there was only good old Pepto Bismol? Do you remember when you helped your mother all day Monday? It was "wash day". Do you remember how good the sheets smelled Monday night, fresh from being on the clothes line all day? Can you remember putting away the "clothes props"?

Do you remember a time when it was okay to be without: without milk in the house, without toothpaste in the bathroom? Did your mother tell you to use the baking soda? Do you remember when we made a list and we shopped once a week? There was no running to the store for the luxuries we have come to call necessities. Isn't it interesting that we "run" to the store? Why don't we say we're going slowly to the store?

Do you remember when there were no magic ice cubes in the refrigerator door? There were no ice cubes at all if someone forgot to refill the ice cube tray!

Can you remember when water quenched your thirst? Coke and Pepsi and Vernor's Ginger Ale were special treats. Why are our mailboxes filled, yet we seem to get no mail?

We were promised free, relaxing time. The TV dinner, the microwave oven, the dryer: they all promised us an easier time. They promised us time to enjoy life, time to relax, time free of stress. They promised us time for the pursuit of happiness.

When I became ill with cancer, I became much more aware that some people are happy and some people are unhappy and, of course, there are those in between. It was then that I began to observe happiness more closely.

I found that happy people seem to breed happy people; that happy teachers have happy students, happy doctors have happy patients, and happy attorneys have happy clients. Happy husbands have happy wives and happy children usually have happy parents.

I found that gentleness, peace, simplicity, forgiveness, humor, trust, fearlessness, and the ability to concentrate seem to make up the happy person. Happy people are "now" people.

Happiness becomes much easier once we realize that it starts with a strong, whole, peaceful state of mind. It then gently extends outward. It is an internal thing. It is not at the mall, in a new, fast car or with the best looking man or woman in the room.

As cancer patients, we were happy. We were willing to take risks. We continued to build competencies and to grow intellectually, aesthetically, spiritually, physically and perceptually. We knew that it was important that we set limits for ourselves.

During my teaching years at Kent State University in the 70's, we went through the love era. Love. Love. Love. Express yourself. Peace and love: that was all we needed.

In the 80's we backed away a little. People like Bruno Bethleheim began saying: "Love is not enough."

A good parent, a good teacher, a good friend does more than simply love. A good tennis player needs more than a love for tennis. A good chef needs more than the love of food.

Our first mission to becoming happier people is the realization that we must believe we have the right to be happy. We then must surround ourselves with happy people and try to look at the world the way we look at children. We must work to enjoy the present and convince ourselves that nothing has to go right to be happy.

Being happy isn't all that hard. Letting go of the unhappiness is probably the most difficult part of the process.

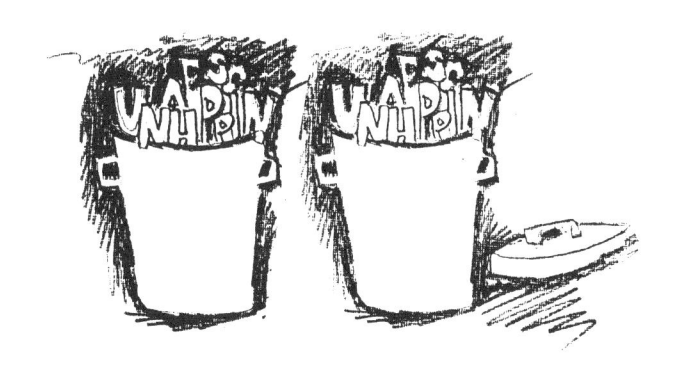

AMAZING GRACE

Growing up in Canton, Ohio, in the 1950's brings back memories of a family of four. We lived in a small, white frame house on a neat, tidy street. The events of each day were pretty predictable. Right, wrong, good, bad were all clearly defined. There were no gray areas. People were in neat, clean categories. Neighborhoods were well defined. Boundaries were clearly set.

We were in the Irish parish. The German parish was just one block away. We played on our own playground. "Those kids" a block away were off limits. There was no doubt in our minds what was expected of us. Rules were laid down. Times were set. Children were to be seen and not heard.

Often I remember feeling guilty because I wondered why. I knew it was wrong for me to ask questions. Why couldn't I wait for the bus at the bus stop a block away from the one beside my school? What were "those kids" a block away like, I wondered?

High school brought six or seven elementary schools together. Kids from the German parish and others from the Italian parish and even some from the Hungarian section of town were in our class. What fun it was to see them. I examined them closely. They weren't any different from me. Yet, I knew that I was permitted to date some, but not others. Why? When I got brave enough to ask, I was told that children weren't supposed to ask questions about things like that. I wanted to be an obedient child.

The Fall of 1955, I entered a state university. I was an art major. I was free. There were all kinds of people; people from different cities, different states, even different countries. My fellow students were of a variety of faiths. I found my own spiritual grounding safe and sound. Others from different faiths were fascinating to me. We spent hours sharing our beliefs. Our first philosophy class energized me.

Someplace along the way, I joined a sorority. It seemed like the thing to do. Others were doing it. Once in, for whatever reason, I rose to the top. Suddenly, I found myself as its president. During a "discussion for membership meeting", to my surprise I learned that one of the young ladies I liked and wanted to invite to join us was not acceptable. Why, I asked? And, I quickly learned from our advisor, who ruled with an iron hand, that Barbara was not of the right faith. I couldn't believe what I heard. Here I was in this new, wide, wonderful world of differences and still there were rigid rules. People were divided into neat little groups. I turned in my tiny gold pin with the tiny gold gavel hanging from its tiny gold chain.

The Summer of 1956, I boarded a train in Cleveland, Ohio, and headed for Lake Placid, New York, to work as a waitress in the vacation spot in the heart of the Adirondack Mountains. The old train chugged along to Buffalo, New York. On the worn maroon mohair seat beside me was a young black girl. We shyly greeted one another. It didn't take long for us to become friends. She told me that she was a Baptist. I had never known a Baptist before. She told me about her grandmama, black-eyed peas, and a delightful life about which I knew nothing. I learned that she too knew about Matthew, Mark, Luke and John. She knew the song **Amazing Grace**. Different faiths, same beliefs. As my world widened, my own spirituality grew deeper. God loved us all.

Several hours into our trip on the train, a stout black man wearing a navy blue uniform and a hat shaped like a pillbox with a black patent leather bill walked through our car.

He announced in litany, "Club car is open. Club car is open. Club car is open."

When I suggested to my new friend that we go to the club car for a cold drink, she told me to go ahead without her. She was not permitted in the club car. She told me that Negroes were not permitted in the club car.

"Why?" I asked.

"That's just the way it is," she said.

My world was getting bigger, but as it got bigger, it got stranger. The stout black man in the navy blue uniform and a hat shaped like a pillbox with a black patent leather bill told of the club car being open, but it wasn't open to everyone.

My first teaching experience was in a school system where we celebrated Yom Kippur and Hanukkah. My students broadened my knowledge of spirituality. I became sensitive to the importance of individuality. I took joy in realizing that from whatever tradition our individual faith comes, it is a part of who we are.

Getting really sick made me aware of the strength of my faith in God. I learned that I respected and appreciated my beliefs and the beliefs of others. I have saved this story until now because it was important that you know me before I shared this part of myself with you. It is important that, as you complete this book, you understand how important my faith and the individual faith of my fellow cancer patients was to us during our illness. It did much to support and give us renewed courage.

I am timid about writing this part of my story because I do not want to be narrow or rigid. The memories of a "right, wrong, good, bad" childhood remain imprinted on my mind.

Cancer fortified and enhanced our spirituality. My love for God was intensified. He was everywhere. He was part of the people I knew and the world that surrounded me. Cancer made my faith in God real. It made me know myself better. It defined what I believed. It gave me peace. Death was never the enemy. It became my friend.

One afternoon while I was meditating in the small chapel our Jesuit priest had carefully prepared for us, I found myself receptive and even anxious about what might be the result of my disease. That day I decided that perhaps

God loved me so much He was calling me to His heavenly home. While my journey had been short, my reason for being was to be accomplished.

What, at one time, would have reduced me to fear and unhappiness brought me love and joy. God drew from His creatures in the presence of the Cross. God was glorified in my illness.

Matthew, Mark, Luke and John became friends. Paul's letters seemed written to me. God showed us Himself. We were brought together in our faiths. Early questions of my youth concerning faith were answered.

Amazing Grace hummed by the young black girl who sat beside me on the worn, maroon mohair train seat in 1956 on our way to Buffalo, New York, echoed in my ears. The experience of God clearly became real. I understood the lessons taught me by the Jewish students about the menorah, Yom Kippur, their Bar Mitzvahs and Bat Mitzvahs. The wonders of our faith sustained and strengthened us. We appreciated one another's way of expressing spirituality.

We did not know tomorrow before cancer. We did not know tomorrow with cancer. Our faith gave us the good sense to turn it over to an all-knowing God. To put it all in His hands felt good. He loved us.

It was to be His will. His will became my will. I was able to relax in the knowledge that He had a plan. He was in control. My job was to listen carefully and follow his instructions.

"I go before you in the sign of faith," He told us.

I looked forward to the future, whatever it was to be. I cherished and enjoyed each day. I looked forward to doing His will. I wanted Him to be glorified in my illness.

Today I appreciate faith in its broadest sense. I enjoy a world with gray areas. Mine is not to judge but to be judged. If I am turned on to God, He will be turned on to me. I see no rigid lines between neighborhoods, parishes, churches, ethnic backgrounds, or colors of skin. Serious illness is binding. It opens our eyes to what is really important in our lives.

As people of faith, we grow even during the darkest of times because out of the darkness will come the light of the Eternal.

CONCLUSION

My story of my journey to wellness has come to an end. I have enjoyed sharing my walk down the path of cancer with you. These 18 years have been full, productive years filled with the hope and happiness of life.

I am glad I waited to write these stories until now. Somehow I lived each one again as I told them to you. Time has sealed and cemented them in my mind. They are stories of reality — the reality of life. They are stories of love and hope, and stories of how strangers become friends and how we really do care for and about one another with real tenderness.

I hope I have informed you and brightened your spirit. I hope I have given you a lift, and even made you laugh. While it is has been my desire to enlighten and educate, I hope each of you realize that the disease cancer can heighten our concept of the beauty of life. Even when we are very, very sick, we can be joyful.

It doesn't matter what our physical condition is as we walk the path of life. It's only important that we not stray from our path to eternal life and that we keep sight of our destination. To focus on the positive is to focus on our eternity. There, and only there, will we reach the perfection we so strongly desire.

My story is not unique. I have just been able to reduce it to writing. There are thousands of stories like mine. Because every man's death diminishes each of us, I addressed the issue of cancer because it very certainly affects today's world. Nothing plays havoc with the balance of the family and questions the very reasons for being than does cancer. The souls of the persons involved are searched for meaning. The sudden changes of everyday routines are quick to shake the stability of even the strongest relationships. Family members are asked to solve problems, to answer questions and to make decisions for which they are inexperienced. These decisions need quick and rational thinking.

Have we been lulled into complacency or does the majority of society know that one of every three persons alive today will eventually be a cancer victim? Cancer is of epidemic proportion. I have attempted to address this issue with assertiveness and sincerity.

Billions of dollars are budgeted yearly to fight our most dreaded enemy. My community role as a cancer research patient at the National Cancer Institute educated and alerted me to devastating effects cancer has on the family. Cancer poses a disruption in family and social relationships. Marriages break up. Family members become angry and then guilty about their anger because of the burden the disease places on them.

Months at The National Institutes of Health in Bethesda, Maryland, for surgery, linear radiation and experimental chemotherapy followed by monthly and now yearly visits, heightened my perception of the outstanding care and dedicated concern of our governmental system in its aggressive attacks on the illness of cancer.

One day during my struggle to get well, I was lying on a table in a small x-ray room. In the adjoining restroom was a twelve year old boy who had had his leg amputated approximately six months earlier because of a sarcoma tumor. Patient privacy and dignity are of utmost importance, but at the same time, rooms are seldom left empty. Time and space are money.

As I waited for the radiologist to adjust the machine, I overheard the soliloquy of this young adult as he attempted to dress his disfigured body. He fought with himself and his world. My heart broke at his awkward attempts to manage this everyday task we all take for granted. His fragile body bumped against the door.

He spoke angrily to himself, "I'm sick of this place, sick of people sticking needles in me, sick of them saying, 'Tomorrow you'll feel better'. I know what tomorrow will be like, another day without my leg, another day of people feeling sorry for me, another day of looking in the mirror at you, the 'you' I hate."

Tears ran down my cheeks as he expressed his anger so eloquently. His recitation was one I'll never forget, one almost too private to repeat. I watched the tormented face of his young, tall, refined mother as she waited for him to complete his chore, one with which he would not allow her to help. The agony and sadness seemed unreal to me. It seemed to take this proud, young person forever to complete a task that at one time took only moments. How must his anger have affected his family? Their energy must have been extinguished in just not being able to help.

Hopefully, today, because of the ongoing research, other young mothers and their sons will not have to witness this agony.

I am alive today because of the care and concern of the people of our country who give of their time and their energy, and because of a governmental agency that carefully uses every cent it is allocated.

My body represents well over three quarters of a million dollars spent in cancer research. These dollars are your tax dollars. Years ago television gave us a make-believe Six Million Dollar Man who could leap over buildings. The National Cancer Institute, funded with your tax dollars, presents you with a real three quarters of a million dollar woman who leaps with joy!

God so loved me that he brought me serenity to cope with the daily business of cancer. He walked with me through the maze of the powerful medical system. He kept my mind sharp and my spirits high. Our Creator has quiet plans for our lives. We live out those plans. I smiled when I was sad for there was always hope. I enjoyed each day and I sometimes had to pretend to understand. I was never a stranger. I never felt lost.

I work to fulfill my dreams so that God can fulfill the dreams He has for me. This is the day that the Lord has made, let us rejoice and be glad as the search for a cure for cancer continues.

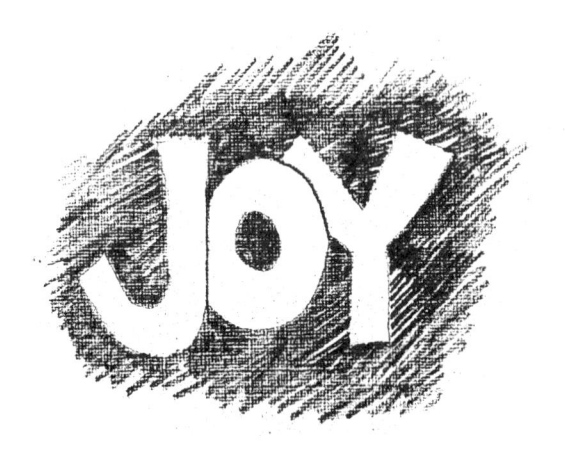

"No one is useless in this world who lightens the burden of anyone else."

Charles Dickens